Renal Diet Cookbook
for
Beginners

Ella Sweetwell

1. Introduction

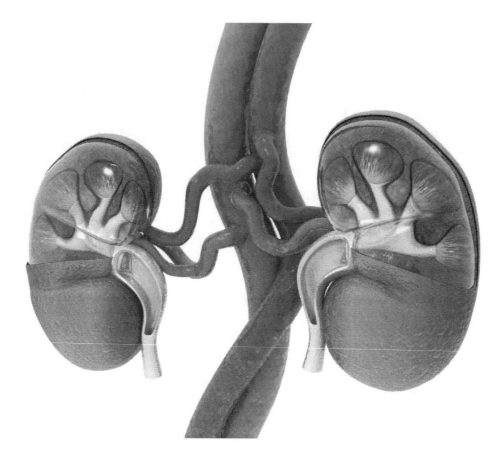

1.1. Understanding Kidney Health

Welcome to the first step in your journey toward managing kidney health through diet. Before diving into the specifics of the renal diet, it's essential to understand the role of your kidneys and how they contribute to your overall health. This knowledge will lay the foundation for everything else in this cookbook.

The Role of Your Kidneys

Your kidneys are two bean-shaped organs, each about the size of a fist, located just below the rib cage on either side of your spine. They perform several critical functions in the body, including:

> **Filtering Waste and Excess Fluids**: Every day, your kidneys filter about 120 to 150 quarts of blood to produce about 1 to 2 quarts of urine, composed of waste and extra fluid.

> **Maintaining Electrolyte Balance**: They regulate the body's balance of electrolytes, such as potassium, phosphorus, and sodium, which are vital for the proper functioning of your muscles, nerves, and other body systems.

> **Producing Hormones**: Your kidneys produce hormones that help regulate blood pressure, make red blood cells, and ensure bone health.

The Impact of Diet on Kidney Health

Diet plays a pivotal role in kidney health for several reasons:

> **Nutrient Management**: Certain nutrients, particularly sodium, potassium, and phosphorus, can accumulate in the body when kidney function is compromised, leading to serious health issues. Managing these through diet is crucial.

> **Protein Processing**: While protein is a vital nutrient, excessive amounts can strain the kidneys. A balance needs to be struck, especially in individuals with kidney disease.

> **Fluid Balance**: In advanced stages of kidney disease, managing fluid intake becomes essential to prevent fluid overload, which can cause swelling, hypertension, and heart strain.

The Importance of a Renal Diet

A renal diet is designed to lessen the workload on the kidneys, helping to slow the progression of kidney disease, manage symptoms, and improve overall health. By carefully choosing foods that support kidney function and limit harmful nutrient accumulation, individuals with kidney disease can significantly impact their health outcomes.

This diet not only focuses on what to avoid but also on what to consume for optimal kidney health. It's tailored to individual needs, taking into account the stage of kidney disease and other health factors, such as the presence of diabetes or high blood pressure.

Understanding your kidney health and the critical role diet plays in supporting it is the first step toward a healthier you. With this foundation, you'll be better equipped to navigate the renal diet, making informed choices that contribute to your well-being. Let's embark on this journey together, with each step bringing you closer to managing your kidney health through thoughtful, nutritious choices.

1.2. Purpose of the Renal Diet

Understanding the rationale behind the renal diet is crucial for anyone embarking on the journey of managing kidney health through nutrition. This diet isn't just about restriction; it's a proactive approach to support your kidneys, enhance your well-being, and potentially slow the progression of kidney disease.

Managing Kidney Disease

The renal diet is specifically tailored to lessen the kidneys' workload, providing them with a break from the high demands of processing certain nutrients. This is particularly important because, as kidney function declines, the body's ability to filter and eliminate waste products and excess fluids diminishes. By adjusting your intake of specific nutrients, you're directly impacting the amount of work your kidneys need to do, which can help in managing kidney disease and preserving kidney function for as long as possible.

Preventing Disease Progression

One of the renal diet's key roles is to help prevent the progression of kidney disease. By carefully managing your diet, you can help control the accumulation of waste products and fluids in your body, reducing the risk of complications associated with kidney disease, such as high blood pressure, bone disease, and heart disease. A well-managed diet can slow the progression of kidney disease, potentially delaying the need for dialysis or kidney transplantation.

Nutrient Focus

The renal diet focuses on several key nutrients:

Sodium: Reducing sodium intake helps control blood pressure, reducing the strain on your kidneys and lowering the risk of cardiovascular disease.

Potassium: Managing potassium levels is crucial, as high levels can lead to dangerous heart rhythms. Kidneys help balance potassium, and impaired kidney function can cause levels to rise.

Phosphorus: High phosphorus levels can cause bone problems and calcification of tissues. The renal diet helps manage phosphorus intake to protect bone health.

Protein: While essential, excessive protein can increase the kidneys' workload. The renal diet often includes moderate protein intake, tailored to individual needs based on the stage of kidney disease.

Fluid Intake

For individuals with advanced kidney disease or those on dialysis, managing fluid intake becomes a critical aspect of the renal diet. Proper fluid management can prevent fluid overload, which can lead to swelling, high blood pressure, and heart issues.

Personalization is Key

It's important to note that the renal diet is not one-size-fits-all. Individual needs can vary significantly based on the stage of kidney disease, presence of other health conditions, and overall nutritional requirements. Consulting with healthcare professionals, including dietitians who specialize in kidney disease, is essential to tailor the diet to your specific needs.

The Goal: A Balanced Approach

The ultimate goal of the renal diet is to maintain optimal health through a balanced approach to nutrition, tailored to support kidney function. By managing key nutrients and making informed food choices, individuals with kidney disease can enjoy a varied, nutritious diet that supports their health and quality of life. This proactive approach empowers individuals to take an active role in managing their kidney health and potentially slowing the progression of kidney disease.

1.3. Who This Book Is For

The "Renal Diet Cookbook for Beginners" is designed to serve as a guiding light for a diverse group of individuals, each at different stages of their journey with kidney health. Whether you've recently been diagnosed with kidney disease, are at risk due to various factors, or simply seek to maintain optimal kidney health, this book offers valuable insights, guidance, and recipes to support your goals.

For Those Newly Diagnosed with Kidney Disease

Receiving a diagnosis of kidney disease can feel overwhelming, with many new terms, dietary restrictions, and lifestyle adjustments to consider. This book aims to simplify this transition, offering easy-to-understand explanations, practical advice, and kidney-friendly recipes that do not compromise on flavor. It's a resource to help you navigate this new phase of your life with confidence and ease.

Individuals at Risk for Kidney Disease

Certain conditions increase the risk of developing kidney disease, including diabetes, hypertension, obesity, and a family history of kidney issues. If you fall into this category, adopting a renal-friendly diet can be a proactive step towards protecting your kidney health. This book provides the tools and knowledge to make dietary choices that can help prevent or delay the onset of kidney disease.

Those Seeking to Maintain Good Kidney Health

Even if you're not at immediate risk or haven't been diagnosed with kidney disease, maintaining kidney health is crucial for overall well-being. The kidneys play a vital role in filtering waste, balancing electrolytes, and regulating blood pressure. This book offers dietary guidelines and recipes that support healthy kidney function, contributing to a balanced and nutritious lifestyle.

Caregivers and Family Members

Caregivers and family members of individuals with kidney disease or those at risk can also benefit from this book. It offers insights into preparing meals that cater to the specific needs of loved ones, making it easier to support their health journey. Sharing meals is a powerful way to offer support, and this book ensures that dietary restrictions don't have to limit the enjoyment and communal aspect of eating.

Health Enthusiasts

Anyone interested in a healthy diet will find this book beneficial. The recipes and guidelines focus on fresh, nutrient-dense ingredients and moderate amounts of key nutrients, aligning well with principles of a balanced, healthy diet. Adopting some of these kidney-friendly eating habits can contribute to overall health and well-being.

In Conclusion

The "Renal Diet Cookbook for Beginners" goes beyond being just a cookbook; it's an all-encompassing guide for those interested in kidney health, whether it's for personal reasons, caregiving, or a healthier lifestyle. It offers foundational knowledge for informed food choices supporting kidney health, paired with tasty recipes making a renal diet both healthy and enjoyable.

2. Fundamentals of the Renal Diet

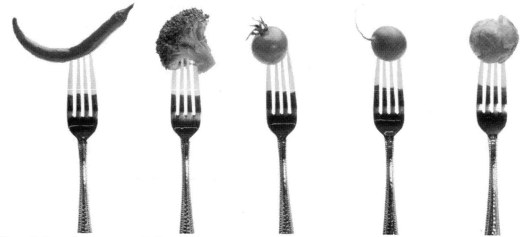

2.1. Key Nutrients to Monitor

When managing kidney health through diet, it's crucial to understand the role of certain nutrients and why their intake needs to be monitored. The renal diet focuses on controlling the intake of sodium, potassium, phosphorus, and protein, as imbalances in these can have significant impacts on kidney function and overall health.

Sodium

Sodium plays a vital role in maintaining fluid balance, nerve function, and muscle contractions. However, when kidney function is compromised, the body may struggle to eliminate excess sodium, leading to fluid retention, high blood pressure, and an increased risk of heart disease.

Recommendations:

Aim for a low-sodium diet, typically less than 2,000 milligrams per day, depending on individual health and stage of kidney disease.

Read food labels carefully to identify hidden sources of sodium.

Opt for fresh, unprocessed foods over canned or processed items, and use herbs and spices instead of salt to flavor meals.

Potassium

Potassium is essential for heart function, muscle contraction, and nerve signaling. While normal kidney function helps maintain proper potassium levels, reduced kidney function can lead to high potassium levels in the blood, a condition known as hyperkalemia. This can cause dangerous heart rhythms and affect muscle function.

Recommendations:

Depending on the stage of kidney disease, a potassium-restricted diet may be necessary.

High-potassium foods, such as bananas, oranges, potatoes, and tomatoes, may need to be limited or avoided.

Consult with a healthcare professional to determine your specific potassium requirements.

Phosphorus

Phosphorus plays a critical role in bone health, energy production, and cell membrane integrity. Kidneys help regulate phosphorus levels, but when kidney function declines, phosphorus can build up in the blood, leading to bone and cardiovascular issues.

Recommendations:

Limit foods high in phosphorus, including dairy products, nuts, seeds, and certain meats.

Phosphorus from animal sources is more easily absorbed by the body than phosphorus found in plant sources, so plant-based options may be preferable for those needing to control phosphorus intake.

Phosphate additives found in processed foods can significantly contribute to phosphorus intake and should be avoided.

Protein

Protein is essential for growth, repair, and maintenance of body tissues. However, a diet high in protein can increase the kidneys' workload, potentially accelerating the progression of kidney disease.

Recommendations:

A moderate-protein diet may be recommended, depending on the stage of kidney disease and individual health needs.

High-quality protein sources, such as lean meats, fish, poultry, and plant-based proteins, should be prioritized.

It's important to balance protein intake with other nutritional needs, ensuring protein consumption supports overall health without overburdening the kidneys.

Implementing the Recommendations

Adjusting your diet to manage these key nutrients involves careful planning and monitoring. Working with a healthcare professional, such as a dietitian specialized in kidney health, can help tailor dietary choices to your specific needs and health status. By controlling the intake of sodium, potassium, phosphorus, and protein, you can significantly contribute to the management of kidney health and overall well-being.

2.2. Reading Food Labels

Navigating food choices on a renal diet becomes much easier with the skill of reading and understanding food labels. This guide aims to demystify the information presented on labels, helping you make informed decisions that align with your dietary needs. Here's what you need to know:

Understanding the Nutrition Facts Panel

The Nutrition Facts panel on packaged foods is your go-to resource for making kidney-friendly choices. Here are the key components to focus on:

> **Serving Size**: Always check the serving size first. All the nutritional information listed is based on this amount. It's crucial for understanding how much of each nutrient you'll consume if you eat one serving, or if you consume more or less than what's considered a serving.

> **Sodium**: Look for the sodium content per serving. Managing sodium intake is vital for controlling blood pressure and reducing the risk of fluid retention. Opt for foods with less than 140 milligrams of sodium per serving, which are considered low sodium.

> **Potassium and Phosphorus**: Not all food labels list potassium and phosphorus, but when they do, it's essential information for those on a renal diet. Your goal should be to manage your intake according to the limits set by your healthcare provider, aiming to avoid high-potassium and high-phosphorus foods if necessary.

Ingredients List

The ingredients list is equally important, as it provides insight into the presence of nutrients that may not be fully detailed in the Nutrition Facts panel.

> **Phosphorus and Potassium**: These elements may not always be listed in the nutritional facts, but their presence can often be inferred from the ingredients. For example, ingredients with "phos" in their names are phosphorus compounds. Similarly, potassium-based additives (like potassium chloride) are indicators of potassium content.

Added Sugars and Salt: Ingredients are listed in order of quantity, from highest to lowest. Watch out for added sugars and salt, especially in the first few ingredients, as these can impact overall health and kidney function.

Identifying Healthy Choices

When managing a renal diet, aim to select foods that are:

Low in sodium: Preferably under 140 mg per serving.

Moderate in potassium and phosphorus, unless otherwise advised by your healthcare professional.

Free from phosphorus additives and high in natural, whole-food ingredients.

Tips for Reading Labels

Be Sodium-Savvy: Remember, "unsalted" doesn't mean sodium-free. Always check the Nutrition Facts.

Watch for Hidden Phosphorus: Phosphorus additives are common in processed foods and do not have to be listed under the nutritional facts. Reading ingredients carefully can help avoid unwanted phosphorus.

Prioritize Whole Foods: Whole, unprocessed foods are generally safer choices for a renal diet, as they naturally contain less sodium, and their potassium and phosphorus content are often more manageable for your body to process.

2.3. Foods to Enjoy vs. Foods to Avoid

When following a renal diet, understanding which foods to embrace and which to limit or avoid is crucial for maintaining optimal kidney health and managing disease progression. This chapter provides comprehensive lists to guide your dietary choices, tailored to support your renal health.

Foods to Enjoy

FRUIT
Apples

Berries (strawberries, blueberries, raspberries)

Grapes

Pineapple

Plums

GRAINS

White rice

Buckwheat

Bulgar (in moderation)

Pasta (refined, not whole grain)

DAIRY AND DAIRY ALTERNATIVES

Rice milk (not enriched)

Almond milk (watch for added phosphorus in ingredients)

Small portions of hard cheese

PROTEIN SOURCES

Egg whites

Skinless chicken

Fish (cod, salmon, tilapia)

Lean cuts of beef

FATS
Olive oil

Avocado (in small amounts due to potassium content)

Unsalted butter

VEGETABLES
Cauliflower

Garlic

Onions

Red bell peppers

Summer squash

Cabbage

Foods to Limit or Avoid

FRUIT
Bananas

Oranges

Orange juice

Kiwi

Avocado (limit to small portions)

Dried fruits

GRAINS
Whole wheat bread and pasta

Bran cereals

Quinoa (high in phosphorus)

PROTEIN SOURCES
Processed meats (bacon, sausage, deli meats)

Nuts and seeds

Beans and lentils (limit or avoid based on potassium content)

DIARY
Milk

Yogurt

Ice cream

Processed cheese

MISCELLANEOUS
Salt and salty seasonings

Prepackaged meals and snacks

Soft drinks

Energy drinks

Chocolate

VEGETABLES
Potatoes and sweet potatoes (unless leached)

Tomatoes and tomato sauce

Spinach

Swiss chard

Beet greens

General Guidelines

Sodium: Aim for foods that are naturally low in sodium or are labeled "no salt added" or "low sodium." Avoid adding salt during cooking or at the table.

Potassium: Be mindful of high-potassium foods, especially fruits and vegetables. Your healthcare provider may recommend specific limits based on your kidney function.

Phosphorus: Avoid foods with added phosphorus, found in many processed foods. Look for "phos" in the ingredient list as an indicator of added phosphorus.

Fluids: Depending on your stage of kidney disease, you may need to monitor your fluid intake. This includes not just water, but also soups, beverages, and foods high in water content.

Conclusion

Adhering to a renal diet by choosing kidney-friendly foods and avoiding those that may harm kidney function is a vital part of managing kidney health. These lists are starting points, and individual dietary needs can vary. Consulting with a healthcare professional, such as a dietitian specialized in renal diets, is crucial to tailor dietary choices to your specific health needs and kidney function status.

3. Getting Started

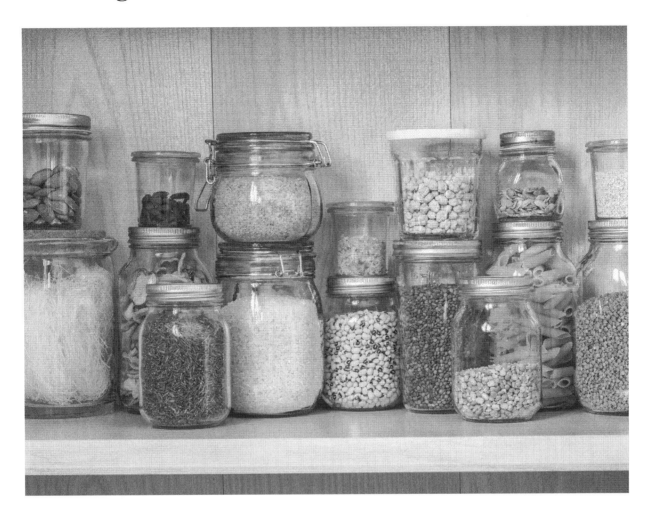

Chapter 3.1: Setting Up Your Kitchen

Transitioning to a renal diet doesn't just involve changing what you eat—it also means rethinking how you stock and organize your kitchen. Having the right ingredients and tools at your disposal can make preparing kidney-friendly meals easier and more enjoyable. Here's how to set up your kitchen to support your renal diet.

Stocking Your Pantry with Renal Diet-Friendly Ingredients

A well-stocked pantry is your first line of defense in sticking to a renal diet. Focus on ingredients that are low in sodium, potassium, and phosphorus, and that can serve as the base for a variety of meals.

Grains and Cereals
- White rice, basmati rice, or jasmine rice
- Pasta made from refined flour (avoid whole grains if phosphorus control is necessary)
- Rice noodles

- Corn tortillas

Canned Goods
- Low or no-sodium canned vegetables
- Unsalted canned beans (rinse thoroughly to remove any added sodium)
- Tuna or salmon packed in water

Condiments and Seasonings

- Fresh or dried herbs and spices (without added salt)
- Vinegar (apple cider, rice, balsamic)
- Lemon and lime juice for flavoring
- Olive oil or other unsaturated oils for cooking and dressings

Snacks

- Unsalted popcorn
- Rice cakes
- Low-sodium crackers

Refrigerator Basics

Keeping fresh produce and certain perishables on hand will ensure you have the ingredients needed to prepare fresh, healthy meals.

Fruits and Vegetables

- Focus on low-potassium choices like apples, berries, cauliflower, and bell peppers.
- Pre-cut vegetables for convenience, ensuring quick access for snacks and cooking.

Proteins

- Fresh cuts of chicken, turkey, and lean beef
- Fresh fish or frozen options without added sodium
- Egg whites or low-phosphorus egg substitutes

Dairy and Alternatives

- Almond, rice, or soy milk (unenriched)
- Small portions of hard cheese or low-phosphorus cheese alternatives

Essential Kitchen Tools

Having the right tools can simplify the preparation of renal-friendly meals and encourage cooking at home, where you have full control over ingredients.

Non-stick Cookware: Reduces the need for cooking oils and fats.

Steamer Basket: A simple way to prepare vegetables while retaining flavor without added salt.

Rice Cooker: Perfect for cooking not just rice but also other grains with minimal monitoring.

Blender or Food Processor: Ideal for making smoothies, purees, and soups from renal-friendly ingredients.

Spice Grinder: Freshly grinding spices enhances flavor naturally, reducing the need for salt.

Measuring Cups and Spoons: Essential for managing portion sizes and ingredient amounts, especially important for controlling nutrient intake.

Tips for a Kidney-Friendly Kitchen

Label Reading: Get into the habit of reading labels for everything you buy, focusing on sodium, potassium, and phosphorus content.

Meal Prep: Dedicate time each week to meal planning and prep. Having kidney-**friendly meals ready to go can prevent dietary missteps.**

Experiment with Flavors: Explore various herbs, spices, and salt-free seasonings to discover new ways to flavor your food without relying on sodium.

Conclusion

Setting up your kitchen for success on a renal diet involves both stocking it with the right ingredients and equipping it with useful tools. By creating an environment that supports your dietary needs, you'll find it easier to adhere to a kidney-friendly eating plan, ensuring your meals are not only nutritious but also enjoyable. With these adjustments, your kitchen will become a haven for healthy, renal diet-compliant cooking.

Chapter 3.2: Meal Planning and Prep

Adopting a renal diet requires thoughtful meal planning and preparation to ensure your nutritional needs are met while managing kidney health. By incorporating strategic meal planning and prep into your routine, you can make the renal diet both manageable and enjoyable, accommodating personal needs and preferences along the way.

Start with a Plan

Understand Your Nutritional Targets

Begin by understanding your specific dietary restrictions and nutritional needs based on your stage of kidney disease. This includes limits on sodium, potassium, phosphorus, and protein intake. Consulting with a healthcare professional or dietitian can provide you with personalized guidelines.

Create a Weekly Meal Plan

> **Diversify Your Meals**: Plan a variety of meals to ensure a wide range of nutrients and keep your diet interesting. Include breakfasts, lunches, dinners, and snacks.

> **Consider Personal Preferences**: Incorporate favorite foods that fit within your dietary restrictions to make the diet more enjoyable.

> **Plan for Leftovers**: Cooking in batches can save time and ensure you have renal-friendly meals on hand.

Grocery Shopping

> **Make a List**: Based on your meal plan, create a shopping list, categorizing items by department (produce, meats, dairy, etc.) to make your shopping trip more efficient.

> **Read Labels**: Choose low-sodium, low-potassium, and low-phosphorus options. Pay close attention to serving sizes and the total nutrient content.

> **Shop the Perimeter**: Fresh produce, lean meats, and dairy alternatives are often found around the store's perimeter. Processed foods, which can be high in sodium and phosphorus, are typically located in the inner aisles.

Meal Prep Strategies

Batch Cooking

Cook large portions of renal-friendly meals at once, then divide them into individual servings to freeze or refrigerate for later use. This approach is especially useful for busy weeks when cooking daily isn't feasible.

Pre-Cut Vegetables and Fruits

Wash, chop, and store vegetables and fruits after your grocery trip. This makes it easier to assemble meals quickly and increases the likelihood of reaching for a healthy snack.

Pre-Portion Snacks

Create grab-and-go snack bags with renal diet-friendly items like apple slices, carrot sticks, or unsalted crackers to help manage portions and make healthy choices convenient.

Adjusting Meals for Personal Needs and Preferences

> **Substitutions**: Learn to make substitutions for high-sodium, high-potassium, or high-phosphorus ingredients with alternatives that better fit your renal diet. For example, replace tomatoes in recipes with red bell peppers for a similar color and sweetness but with less potassium.

> **Flexible Recipes**: Choose recipes that easily adapt to different dietary needs. For instance, a stir-fry can accommodate various vegetables that meet your nutritional guidelines.

> **Seasoning Without Salt**: Experiment with herbs, spices, lemon juice, and vinegar to add flavor to dishes without increasing sodium content.

Tips for Successful Meal Planning and Prep

> **Stay Organized**: Keep your meal plan, recipes, and shopping list in a visible place, such as on the refrigerator or a digital app, to stay on track.

> **Involve Family Members**: When planning meals, consider the preferences of others in your household. Many renal diet recipes can be adapted to please the whole family by adding or subtracting certain ingredients for individual plates.

> **Regular Review**: Periodically review and adjust your meal plan as your dietary needs, preferences, or routine change.

4. Recipes

Breakfast Recipes

Starting your day with a nutrient-rich, kidney-friendly meal sets a positive tone for the rest of the day, especially when managing kidney health. Breakfast is not just the first meal of the day; it's an opportunity to provide your body with the energy and nutrients it needs to function optimally, while also taking care to not overburden your kidneys.

For those following a renal diet, breakfast becomes an essential component of dietary management. The morning meal is an opportune time to include foods that support kidney health, carefully selected to avoid excess sodium, potassium, phosphorus, and to manage protein intake according to individual dietary needs. It's about finding a balance that nourishes the body without contributing to kidney stress.

Choosing the right ingredients and preparing them in a way that maximizes both flavor and nutritional value is key. This can include incorporating low-potassium fruits, utilizing egg whites or high-quality protein sources that are easier on the kidneys, and selecting grains and cereals that are lower in phosphorus. By doing so, you can create breakfasts that are not only delicious but also align with your nutritional goals.

Moreover, a well-planned renal-friendly breakfast can help maintain stable energy levels throughout the morning, reducing the temptation for unhealthy snacking that might not align with your dietary restrictions. It's also a chance to hydrate with kidney-friendly beverages, setting a positive hydration pattern for the day.

This section of the cookbook is dedicated to providing you with a variety of breakfast recipes designed to meet the criteria of a renal diet without sacrificing taste or satisfaction. Whether you prefer a quick and easy meal to grab on the go or have the time to savor a more leisurely breakfast, these recipes are crafted to ensure that you start your day in the healthiest, most delicious way possible.

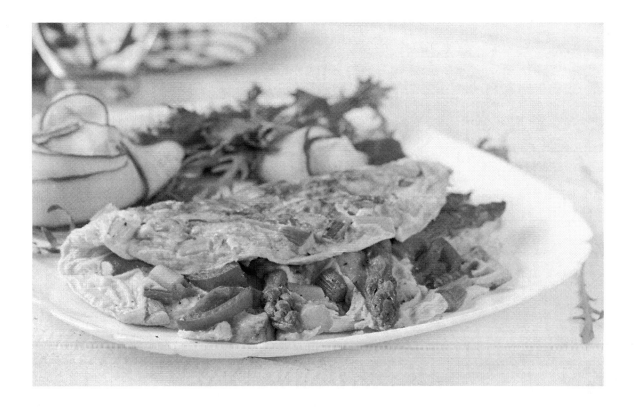

Low Sodium Omelet: A Protein-Rich Start with Lots of Vegetables

Preparation Time: 10 min | Cooking Time: 5 min | Serving Size: 1 omelet

Ingredients

- 3 egg whites or ½ cup low-phosphorus egg substitute
- ¼ cup diced red bell peppers
- ¼ cup diced green bell peppers
- ¼ cup chopped spinach
- 2 tablespoons chopped onions
- 1 tablespoon olive oil
- Fresh herbs (such as parsley or chives), for garnish
- Black pepper, to taste

Step-by-Step Cooking Instructions

Prep the Vegetables: Dice the bell peppers and chop the spinach and onions finely to ensure they cook quickly and evenly.

Heat the Skillet: Warm the olive oil in a non-stick skillet over medium heat. Add the onions and bell peppers, sautéing until they are soft, about 3-5 minutes.

Add Spinach: Toss in the chopped spinach and cook until it wilts, approximately 1-2 minutes. Remove the vegetables from the skillet and set aside.

Cook the Egg Whites: In the same skillet, pour in the egg whites or egg substitute. Cook without stirring for a few seconds until they begin to set around the edges.

Fill the Omelet: Sprinkle the sautéed vegetables evenly over one half of the omelet. Continue cooking until the eggs are set but still slightly runny on top.

Fold and Serve: Carefully fold the omelet in half, covering the vegetables. Let it cook for another minute. Garnish with fresh herbs and black pepper. Serve hot.

Sodium: Approximately 70mg | Potassium: Approximately 200mg | Phosphorus: Approximately 60mg | Protein: Approximately 14g

This Low Sodium Omelet not only meets the dietary restrictions of a renal diet but also proves that eating healthily doesn't have to mean sacrificing flavor or variety.

Renal-Friendly Pancakes

Preparation Time: 15 min | Cooking Time: 10 min | Serving Size: 2 pancakes

Ingredients

- 1 cup all-purpose flour
- 1 tablespoon sugar
- 2 teaspoons low-phosphorus leavening agent (calcium acid phosphate-based baking powder)
- ½ cup low-phosphorus egg substitute or 2 egg whites
- ¾ cup almond milk or rice milk
- 2 tablespoons unsalted butter, melted
- 1 teaspoon vanilla extract
- Fresh berries or low-potassium fruits for topping

Step-by-Step Cooking Instructions

Mix Dry Ingredients: In a large bowl, whisk together the flour, sugar, and low-phosphorus baking powder.

Combine Wet Ingredients: In another bowl, mix the egg substitute or egg whites, almond or rice milk, melted butter, and vanilla extract until well combined.

Combine Wet and Dry: Gradually pour the wet ingredients into the dry, mixing until just combined to avoid overmixing. The batter should be slightly lumpy.

Preheat the Pan: Heat a non-stick skillet over medium heat and lightly coat with cooking spray.

Cook Pancakes: Pour ¼ cup of batter for each pancake onto the skillet. Cook until bubbles form on the surface, then flip and cook until golden brown on the other side.

Serve: Serve the pancakes warm, topped with fresh berries or low-potassium fruits of your choice.

Sodium: Approximately 100mg | Potassium: Approximately 150mg | Phosphorus: Approximately 100mg | Protein: Approximately 6g

Apple and Cinnamon Porridge

Preparation Time: 5 min | Cooking Time: 15 min | Serving Size: 1 serving

Ingredients

- ½ cup rolled oats
- 1 cup almond milk or rice milk
- 1 medium apple, peeled and diced
- ½ teaspoon cinnamon
- 1 tablespoon honey or maple syrup (optional)
- A pinch of salt (optional)

Step-by-Step Cooking Instructions

Combine Ingredients: In a medium saucepan, combine the rolled oats, almond or rice milk, diced apple, cinnamon, and a pinch of salt (if using). Mix well.
Cook the Porridge: Place the saucepan over medium heat and bring to a simmer. Reduce the heat to low and cook, stirring occasionally, for about 15 minutes, or until the oats are fully cooked and the porridge has thickened to your liking.
Sweeten: Stir in honey or maple syrup (if using) to sweeten the porridge.
Serve: Transfer the porridge to a bowl and serve warm. For an extra touch, top with a sprinkle of cinnamon or additional apple slices.

Sodium: Approximately 30mg | Potassium: Approximately 200mg | Phosphorus: Approximately 150mg | Protein: Approximately 5g

This Apple and Cinnamon Porridge is a warming and nutritious breakfast option, perfect for those following a renal diet. The combination of sweet apple and cinnamon paired with the hearty texture of oats provides a satisfying start to the day while keeping your dietary needs in mind.

Buckwheat Pancakes

Preparation Time: 10 min | Cooking Time: 15 min | Serving Size: 2 pancakes

Ingredients

- 1 cup buckwheat flour
- 1 teaspoon baking powder (low-phosphorus, if available)
- 2 tablespoons honey or maple syrup
- 1 cup almond milk or rice milk
- 1 egg or ¼ cup low-phosphorus egg substitute
- 2 tablespoons melted unsalted butter or coconut oil
- 1 teaspoon vanilla extract
- Cooking spray or additional oil for the pan

Step-by-Step Cooking Instructions

Mix Dry Ingredients: In a large mixing bowl, sift together the buckwheat flour and baking powder.

Combine Wet Ingredients: In another bowl, whisk together the honey or maple syrup, almond or rice milk, egg or egg substitute, melted butter or coconut oil, and vanilla extract until well blended.

Combine Wet and Dry: Gradually pour the wet mixture into the dry ingredients, stirring until just combined. Be careful not to overmix; a few lumps are okay.

Cook the Pancakes: Heat a non-stick skillet or griddle over medium heat and lightly coat with cooking spray or oil. Pour ¼ cup of batter for each pancake onto the skillet. Cook until bubbles appear on the surface and the edges look set, about 2-3 minutes. Flip and cook for an additional 2 minutes or until golden brown.

Serve Warm: Serve the pancakes warm with your choice of toppings, such as fresh fruit or a drizzle of maple syrup.

Sodium: Approximately 50mg | Potassium: Approximately 234mg | Phosphorus: Approximately 118mg | Protein: Approximately 6g

Egg White and Spinach Frittata

Preparation Time: 5 min | Cooking Time: 20 min | Serving Size: 2 servings

Ingredients

- 6 egg whites
- 2 cups fresh spinach, washed and roughly chopped
- 1 small onion, finely diced
- 1 medium tomato, diced
- 1/4 cup shredded low-sodium cheese (optional)
- 1 teaspoon olive oil
- Salt (optional) and pepper to taste
- Fresh herbs (such as parsley or chives) for garnish

Step-by-Step Cooking Instructions

Sauté Vegetables: Heat olive oil in a non-stick, oven-safe skillet over medium heat. Add the onion and sauté until translucent, about 3 minutes. Add the spinach and cook until wilted, about 2 minutes. Stir in the diced tomato and cook for an additional 1 minute.

Prepare Egg Whites: In a bowl, whisk the egg whites with a pinch of salt (optional) and pepper until frothy.

Combine and Cook: Pour the egg whites over the sautéed vegetables in the skillet, ensuring the mixture is evenly spread. Cook over medium heat without stirring, until the edges start to set, about 5 minutes.

Oven Finish: Sprinkle with shredded low-sodium cheese (if using) and transfer the skillet to a preheated oven at 375°F (190°C). Bake until the frittata is set and the top is lightly golden, about 12-15 minutes.

Garnish and Serve: Remove from the oven, let cool slightly, and garnish with fresh herbs. Slice into wedges and serve warm.

Sodium: Approximately 200mg | Potassium: Approximately 340mg | Phosphorus: Approximately 120mg | Protein: Approximately 18g

Vanilla Almond Oatmeal

Preparation Time: 5 min | Cooking Time: 10 min | Serving Size: 1 serving

Ingredients

- ½ cup rolled oats
- 1 cup almond milk
- 1 teaspoon vanilla extract
- 1 tablespoon almond slices
- 1 teaspoon honey or maple syrup (optional)
- A pinch of salt

Step-by-Step Cooking Instructions

Cook Oats: In a small saucepan, bring the almond milk to a low simmer over medium heat. Add the oats and a pinch of salt, stirring occasionally, for about 5 minutes or until the oats are soft and the mixture has thickened.

Add Flavors: Stir in the vanilla extract and honey or maple syrup (if using), mixing well to combine all the flavors.

Serve: Pour the oatmeal into a bowl, top with almond slices, and serve warm.

Nutritional Information per Serving

Sodium: Approximately 80mg | Potassium: Approximately 150mg | Phosphorus: Approximately 200mg | Protein: Approximately 6g

This Vanilla Almond Oatmeal is a simple yet delightful way to start your day, offering a warm and comforting meal that fits within the guidelines of a renal diet. The combination of vanilla and almond provides a subtle sweetness and nuttiness, making it a satisfying breakfast option.

Berry Smoothie Bowl

Preparation Time: 10 min | Cooking Time: 0 min | Serving Size: 1 serving

Ingredients

- 1 cup mixed berries (strawberries, blueberries, raspberries), fresh or frozen
- 1 banana, sliced
- ½ cup almond milk or rice milk
- ¼ cup Greek yogurt (use a low-phosphorus variety if available)
- 1 tablespoon chia seeds
- Optional toppings: sliced almonds, additional berries, a sprinkle of granola (low sodium)

Step-by-Step Cooking Instructions

Blend Smoothie Base: In a blender, combine the mixed berries, banana, almond milk, Greek yogurt, and chia seeds. Blend until smooth and creamy.

Assemble Bowl: Pour the smoothie mixture into a bowl.

Add Toppings: Garnish with your choice of toppings, such as sliced almonds, additional berries, or a sprinkle of granola, keeping in mind the nutritional content of each.

Nutritional Information per Serving

Sodium: Approximately 50mg | Potassium: Approximately 400mg | Phosphorus: Approximately 150mg | Protein: Approximately 8g

This Berry Smoothie Bowl is a vibrant and nutritious breakfast option, combining the natural sweetness and antioxidants of berries with the protein-packed goodness of Greek yogurt and chia seeds. It's a quick and easy meal that fits into a renal-friendly diet, offering a delicious way to start your day with minimal preparation.

Zucchini and Carrot Muffins

Preparation Time: 15 min | Cooking Time: 20 min | Serving Size: 12 muffins

Ingredients

- 1 cup grated zucchini (squeeze out excess moisture)
- 1 cup grated carrot
- 2 cups all-purpose flour
- 1 teaspoon baking powder (low-phosphorus, if available)
- 1/2 teaspoon baking soda
- 1/4 cup unsalted butter, melted
- 1/2 cup honey or maple syrup
- 2 egg whites or 1/2 cup low-phosphorus egg substitute
- 1 teaspoon vanilla extract
- 1/2 teaspoon cinnamon
- A pinch of salt

Step-by-Step Cooking Instructions

Preheat Oven: Preheat your oven to 350°F (175°C). Line a muffin tin with paper liners or lightly grease it.

Combine Dry Ingredients: In a large bowl, whisk together the flour, baking powder, baking soda, cinnamon, and a pinch of salt.

Mix Wet Ingredients: In another bowl, mix the melted butter, honey or maple syrup, egg whites or egg substitute, and vanilla extract until well combined.

Combine Mixtures: Add the wet ingredients to the dry ingredients, stirring until just combined. Fold in the grated zucchini and carrot.

Bake: Spoon the batter into the prepared muffin tin, filling each cup about 3/4 full. Bake for 20 minutes, or until a toothpick inserted into the center of a muffin comes out clean.

Cool: Let the muffins cool in the pan for 5 minutes before transferring them to a wire rack to cool completely.

Sodium: Approximately 55mg | Potassium: Approximately 90mg | Phosphorus: Approximately 60mg | Protein: Approximately 3g

Apple Cinnamon Porridge

Preparation Time: 5 min | Cooking Time: 15 min | Serving Size: 1 serving

Ingredients

- ½ cup rolled oats
- 1 cup water or almond milk
- 1 medium apple, peeled and diced
- ½ teaspoon cinnamon
- 1 tablespoon honey or maple syrup (optional)
- A pinch of salt

Step-by-Step Cooking Instructions

Cook Oats: In a medium saucepan, bring the water or almond milk to a boil. Add the oats and a pinch of salt, then reduce the heat to a simmer.

Add Apple: Stir in the diced apple and cinnamon. Continue to simmer, stirring occasionally, until the oats are soft and the mixture has thickened, about 15 minutes.

Sweeten: Remove from heat and stir in honey or maple syrup, if desired.

Serve Warm: Spoon the porridge into a bowl and serve warm. For added texture and flavor, sprinkle with more cinnamon or top with additional diced apple.

Sodium: Approximately 30mg | Potassium: Approximately 200mg | Phosphorus: Approximately 120mg | Protein: Approximately 3g

This Apple Cinnamon Porridge is a warm and comforting breakfast, perfectly suited for those following a renal diet. It combines the natural sweetness of apples with the heartiness of oats and a hint of cinnamon for a delicious start to your day. Easy to prepare and customize, it's a nutritious meal that supports kidney health.

Vegetable Breakfast Burritos

Preparation Time: 10 min | Cooking Time: 15 min | Serving Size: 2 burritos

Ingredients

- 4 egg whites or ½ cup low-phosphorus egg substitute
- 2 low-sodium whole wheat tortillas
- ½ cup diced bell peppers (any color)
- ¼ cup diced onions
- ½ cup fresh spinach, roughly chopped
- ¼ cup shredded low-sodium cheese (optional)
- 1 tablespoon olive oil
- Salt (optional) and pepper to taste

Step-by-Step Cooking Instructions

Sauté Vegetables: In a non-stick skillet, heat the olive oil over medium heat. Add the diced bell peppers and onions, sautéing until they are soft, about 5 minutes. Add the spinach and cook until wilted, about 2 minutes.

Cook Egg Whites: In another pan or the same pan pushed to one side, pour in the egg whites or egg substitute. Season with a pinch of salt (if using) and pepper. Scramble over medium heat until fully cooked, about 3-4 minutes.

Assemble Burritos: Lay out the whole wheat tortillas on a flat surface. Divide the cooked vegetables and scrambled egg whites evenly between the tortillas. Sprinkle shredded cheese on top if desired.

Roll Burritos: Fold in the sides of each tortilla and roll tightly to enclose the filling. Optionally, you can place the rolled burritos back in the skillet to lightly toast the outside.

Serve Warm: Cut each burrito in half, if desired, and serve warm.

Sodium: Approximately 200mg | Potassium: Approximately 250mg | Phosphorus: Approximately 100mg | Protein: Approximately 12g

Greek Yogurt with Honey and Walnuts

Preparation Time: 5 min | Cooking Time: 0 min | Serving Size: 1 serving

Ingredients

- 1 cup low-fat Greek yogurt
- 1 tablespoon honey
- 2 tablespoons walnuts, chopped

Step-by-Step Cooking Instructions

Combine Ingredients: In a serving bowl, add the Greek yogurt.
Add Honey: Drizzle the honey over the Greek yogurt.
Top with Walnuts: Sprinkle the chopped walnuts on top of the honeyed yogurt.
Serve: Mix lightly before eating, if desired, or enjoy as layered.

Sodium: Approximately 50mg | Potassium: Approximately 240mg | Phosphorus: Approximately 200mg | Protein: Approximately 20g

This Greek Yogurt with Honey and Walnuts is a simple yet decadent breakfast or snack option. It combines the creamy texture of Greek yogurt with the natural sweetness of honey and the crunchy texture of walnuts, providing a balanced meal that's rich in protein and calcium while being mindful of renal dietary restrictions.

Savory Mushroom Toast

Preparation Time: 10 min | Cooking Time: 10 min | Serving Size: 2 toasts

Ingredients

- 4 slices whole-grain bread (low sodium)
- 1 cup sliced mushrooms
- 2 tablespoons olive oil
- 1 clove garlic, minced
- 2 tablespoons low-sodium cheese, grated (optional)
- Salt (optional) and pepper to taste
- Fresh thyme or parsley for garnish

Step-by-Step Cooking Instructions

Sauté Mushrooms: In a skillet, heat the olive oil over medium heat. Add the garlic and sauté for 1 minute. Add the mushrooms, season with pepper (and a pinch of salt, if using), and cook until the mushrooms are tender and browned, about 8 minutes.
Toast Bread: While the mushrooms are cooking, toast the bread slices to your desired crispness.
Assemble Toasts: Spoon the sautéed mushrooms evenly over the toasted bread slices. Sprinkle with low-sodium cheese, if using.
Broil (Optional): For melted cheese, place the mushroom-topped toasts under a broiler for 1-2 minutes or until the cheese is bubbly and golden.
Garnish and Serve: Garnish with fresh thyme or parsley before serving.

Sodium: Approximately 100mg | Potassium: Approximately 150mg | Phosphorus: Approximately 100mg | Protein: Approximately 8g

"Savory Mushroom Toast" is a delightful and nutritious option for those on a renal diet, offering a blend of earthy mushrooms and hearty whole-grain toast. It's perfect for a satisfying breakfast or a wholesome snack.

Lunch Recipes

Lunch plays a crucial role in the daily diet, providing the energy and nutrients needed to maintain focus and performance throughout the afternoon. For those managing kidney health, a fulfilling midday meal is particularly important, as it needs to nourish the body without placing unnecessary strain on the kidneys. The recipes in this section are designed with this balance in mind, offering delicious, kidney-friendly options that are both satisfying and easy to digest.

Each recipe has been carefully crafted to ensure it supports kidney health, focusing on low sodium, controlled potassium and phosphorus levels, and moderate protein content. By incorporating a variety of fresh vegetables, lean proteins, and whole grains, these lunch options will keep you energized and satisfied, without the risk of fatigue or discomfort that can come from heavier meals.

Whether you're at home, at work, or on the go, these lunch recipes provide tasty and practical solutions for staying true to your renal diet. From vibrant salads and hearty soups to flavorful sandwiches and wraps, you'll discover new favorites that make midday meals a highlight of your day. Enjoy the benefits of meals that not only taste great but also contribute positively to your kidney health and overall well-being.

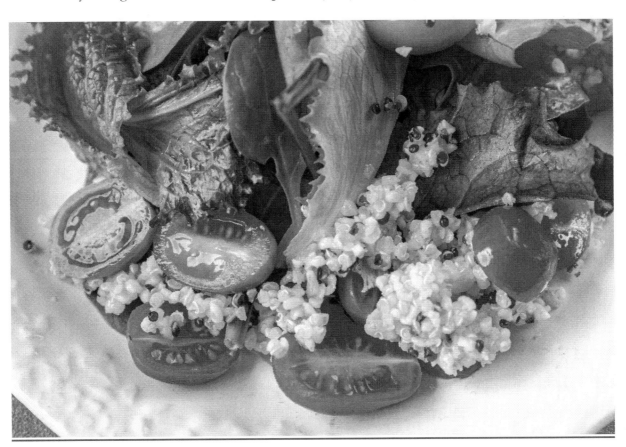

Quinoa Salad with Lemon Vinaigrette

Preparation Time: 15 min | Cooking Time: 20 min | Serving Size: 4 servings

Ingredients

- 1 cup quinoa, rinsed
- 2 cups water
- 1/2 cup diced cucumbers
- 1/2 cup cherry tomatoes, halved
- 1/4 cup finely chopped red onion
- 1/4 cup diced bell peppers (any color)
- 1/4 cup chopped fresh parsley
- 2 tablespoons olive oil
- Juice of 1 lemon
- 1 garlic clove, minced
- Salt (optional) and pepper to taste

Step-by-Step Cooking Instructions

Cook Quinoa: In a medium saucepan, bring 2 cups of water to a boil. Add quinoa, reduce heat to low, cover, and simmer for about 15-20 minutes or until all water is absorbed and quinoa is fluffy.
Prepare Vegetables: While the quinoa is cooking, prepare the cucumbers, cherry tomatoes, red onion, bell peppers, and parsley. Set aside in a large salad bowl.
Make Lemon Vinaigrette: In a small bowl, whisk together olive oil, lemon juice, minced garlic, salt (if using), and pepper until well combined.
Combine: Once the quinoa is cooked and slightly cooled, add it to the salad bowl with the vegetables. Pour the lemon vinaigrette over the salad and toss to combine.
Chill: Refrigerate the salad for at least 30 minutes before serving to allow the flavors to meld.

Sodium: Approximately 30mg | Potassium: Approximately 250mg | Phosphorus: Approximately 150mg | Protein: Approximately 6g

Grilled Chicken Wrap

Preparation Time: 15 min | Cooking Time: 10 min | Serving Size: 2 wraps

Ingredients

- 2 boneless, skinless chicken breasts
- 2 whole wheat tortillas (low sodium)
- 1 cup fresh spinach leaves
- 1/2 red bell pepper, thinly sliced
- 1/4 cup shredded low-sodium cheese (optional)
- 1 tablespoon olive oil
- 1 teaspoon dried oregano
- Salt (optional) and pepper to taste
- 2 tablespoons low-sodium Greek yogurt

Step-by-Step Cooking Instructions

Prep Chicken: Season chicken breasts with olive oil, oregano, salt (if using), and pepper.

Grill Chicken: Grill the chicken over medium heat for about 5 minutes on each side or until fully cooked through. Let it rest for a few minutes, then slice thinly.

Assemble Wraps: Lay out the whole wheat tortillas on a flat surface. Spread 1 tablespoon of Greek yogurt on each tortilla. Divide the spinach leaves and red bell pepper slices evenly among the tortillas.

Add Chicken: Place the grilled chicken slices on top of the vegetables. If using, sprinkle the shredded low-sodium cheese over the chicken.

Roll Wraps: Fold in the sides of the tortillas and roll them tightly to enclose the filling.

Serve: Cut each wrap in half and serve immediately, or wrap in foil to keep warm until serving.

Sodium: Approximately 200mg | Potassium: Approximately 300mg | Phosphorus: Approximately 250mg | Protein: Approximately 25g

Vegetable Soup

Preparation Time: 15 min | Cooking Time: 30 min | Serving Size: 4 servings

Ingredients

- 2 tablespoons olive oil
- 1 medium onion, diced
- 2 cloves garlic, minced
- 2 medium carrots, peeled and diced
- 2 stalks celery, diced
- 1 small zucchini, diced
- 1 cup green beans, trimmed and cut into 1-inch pieces
- 4 cups low-sodium vegetable broth
- 1 (14.5-ounce) can no-salt-added diced tomatoes
- 1 teaspoon dried thyme
- 1 teaspoon dried oregano
- Salt (optional) and pepper to taste
- 1 cup chopped fresh spinach

Step-by-Step Cooking Instructions

Sauté Vegetables: In a large pot, heat the olive oil over medium heat. Add the onion and garlic, sautéing until soft, about 5 minutes. Add the carrots and celery, cooking for another 5 minutes.

Add Remaining Vegetables: Stir in the zucchini and green beans, cooking for a few minutes before adding the vegetable broth, diced tomatoes (with their juice), thyme, and oregano.

Simmer: Bring the soup to a boil, then reduce the heat and let it simmer, uncovered, for about 20 minutes, or until the vegetables are tender.

Final Touches: Add the chopped spinach and cook for an additional 2-3 minutes until the spinach is wilted. Season with salt (if using) and pepper to taste.

Serve: Ladle the soup into bowls and serve warm.

Sodium: Approximately 150mg | Potassium: Approximately 400mg | Phosphorus: Approximately 100mg | Protein: Approximately 4g

Quinoa Salad with Lemon Vinaigrette

Preparation Time: 15 min | Cooking Time: 20 min | Serving Size: 4 servings

Ingredients

- 1 cup quinoa
- 2 cups water
- 1/2 cup diced cucumbers
- 1/2 cup cherry tomatoes, halved
- 1/4 cup finely chopped red onion
- 1/4 cup diced bell peppers
- 1/4 cup chopped fresh parsley
- 2 tablespoons olive oil
- Juice of 1 lemon
- 1 garlic clove, minced
- Salt (optional) and pepper to taste

Step-by-Step Cooking Instructions

Cook Quinoa: In a medium saucepan, bring the quinoa and water to a boil. Reduce heat to low, cover, and simmer until quinoa is tender and water is absorbed, about 15 to 20 minutes. Let cool.

Prepare Vegetables: While quinoa is cooling, dice cucumbers, halve cherry tomatoes, finely chop red onion, dice bell peppers, and chop parsley.

Make Lemon Vinaigrette: In a small bowl, whisk together olive oil, lemon juice, minced garlic, and season with salt (optional) and pepper.

Combine Salad: In a large bowl, combine cooled quinoa, prepared vegetables, and parsley. Pour lemon vinaigrette over the salad and toss to combine.

Chill and Serve: Chill the salad for at least 30 minutes before serving to allow flavors to meld.

Sodium: Approximately 30mg | Potassium: Approximately 250mg | Phosphorus: Approximately 150mg | Protein: Approximately 6g

Turkey and Avocado Wrap

Preparation Time: 10 min | Cooking Time: 0 min | Serving Size: 2 wraps

Ingredients

- 2 whole wheat tortillas (low sodium)
- 4 slices of low-sodium turkey breast
- 1 ripe avocado, sliced
- 1/2 cup shredded lettuce
- 1/4 cup diced tomatoes
- 2 tablespoons low-sodium ranch dressing or Greek yogurt
- Pepper to taste

Step-by-Step Cooking Instructions

Prepare the Wraps: Lay out the whole wheat tortillas on a clean surface.

Layer Ingredients: On each tortilla, evenly distribute the turkey slices, avocado slices, shredded lettuce, and diced tomatoes.

Add Dressing: Drizzle each wrap with 1 tablespoon of low-sodium ranch dressing or Greek yogurt. Add pepper to taste.

Roll the Wraps: Carefully roll each tortilla tightly to enclose the filling. If needed, you can use a toothpick to secure the wrap.

Serve: Cut each wrap in half, if desired, and serve immediately for the freshest taste.

Sodium: Approximately 200mg | Potassium: Approximately 350mg | Phosphorus: Approximately 100mg | Protein: Approximately 15g

This Turkey and Avocado Wrap is a delicious and renal-friendly option for a quick lunch or a light dinner. Packed with lean protein and healthy fats from the avocado, it's a nutritious choice that doesn't compromise on flavor. The whole wheat tortillas provide a good source of fiber while keeping the sodium content low, making this wrap a great addition to a kidney-friendly diet.

Mediterranean-inspired Stuffed Peppers

Preparation Time: 20 min | Cooking Time: 30 min | Serving Size: 4 servings

Ingredients

- 4 large bell peppers, any color
- 1 cup cooked quinoa
- 1/2 cup diced tomatoes, drained
- 1/4 cup crumbled feta cheese (low sodium)
- 1/4 cup chopped black olives
- 1/4 cup diced red onion
- 2 tablespoons chopped fresh parsley
- 2 cloves garlic, minced
- 1 tablespoon olive oil
- Juice of 1 lemon
- Salt (optional) and pepper to taste

Step-by-Step Cooking Instructions

Prep Peppers: Preheat oven to 375°F (190°C). Cut the tops off the bell peppers and remove the seeds. Set aside.

Mix Filling: In a bowl, combine the cooked quinoa, diced tomatoes, feta cheese, black olives, red onion, parsley, and garlic. Drizzle with olive oil and lemon juice, then season with salt (optional) and pepper. Stir until well mixed.

Stuff Peppers: Spoon the quinoa mixture into each bell pepper, pressing down gently to pack.

Bake: Place the stuffed peppers in a baking dish. Cover with foil and bake in the preheated oven for about 25-30 minutes, or until the peppers are tender.

Serve: Remove from oven, let cool slightly, and serve warm.

Sodium: Approximately 150mg | Potassium: Approximately 300mg | Phosphorus: Approximately 120mg | Protein: Approximately 6g

Grilled Chicken Caesar Salad (Low-Sodium Dressing)

Preparation Time: 15 min | Cooking Time: 10 min | Serving Size: 4 servings

Ingredients

- 2 boneless, skinless chicken breasts
- 8 cups romaine lettuce, chopped
- 1/2 cup low-sodium Caesar dressing
- 1/4 cup grated Parmesan cheese (low sodium)
- 1 cup whole grain croutons
- 1 teaspoon olive oil
- Black pepper to taste
- Lemon wedges for garnish

Step-by-Step Cooking Instructions

Grill Chicken: Preheat the grill to medium-high heat. Brush chicken breasts with olive oil and season with black pepper. Grill for 5 minutes on each side or until fully cooked through. Let it rest for a few minutes, then slice thinly.

Prepare Salad: In a large salad bowl, toss the chopped romaine lettuce with the low-sodium Caesar dressing until evenly coated.

Assemble Salad: Add the grilled chicken slices and whole grain croutons to the salad. Toss lightly to combine.

Serve: Divide the salad among plates. Sprinkle with grated Parmesan cheese and garnish with lemon wedges.

Sodium: Approximately 200mg | Potassium: Approximately 300mg | Phosphorus: Approximately 150mg | Protein: Approximately 25g

Vegetable Stir-Fry with Rice

Preparation Time: 15 min | Cooking Time: 20 min | Serving Size: 4 servings

Ingredients

- 2 cups cooked white rice (preferably cooked in low-sodium broth)
- 1 tablespoon olive oil
- 1 cup broccoli florets
- 1/2 cup sliced carrots
- 1/2 cup sliced bell peppers (any color)
- 1/2 cup snow peas
- 1/4 cup low-sodium soy sauce or tamari
- 1 teaspoon grated ginger
- 1 garlic clove, minced
- 1 tablespoon cornstarch mixed with 2 tablespoons water (optional, for thickening)
- 1 teaspoon sesame oil (optional, for flavor)
- Fresh scallions for garnish

Step-by-Step Cooking Instructions

Prep Ingredients: Ensure all vegetables are washed, cut into bite-sized pieces, and rice is cooked ahead of time.

Cook Vegetables: Heat olive oil in a large skillet or wok over medium-high heat. Add broccoli and carrots; stir-fry for about 5 minutes. Add bell peppers and snow peas; continue stir-frying until all vegetables are tender yet crisp, about 3-4 more minutes.

Add Flavor: Stir in the low-sodium soy sauce or tamari, grated ginger, and minced garlic into the skillet. Mix well to evenly coat the vegetables. If using cornstarch mixture, add it now to thicken the sauce.

Combine with Rice: Lower the heat to medium. Add the cooked rice to the skillet with the vegetables, mixing thoroughly until the rice is heated through and all ingredients are well combined.

Final Touch: Drizzle with sesame oil (if using) and toss again. Serve hot, garnished with fresh scallions.

Sodium: Approximately 300mg | Potassium: Approximately 200mg | Phosphorus: Approximately 100mg | Protein: Approximately 5g

Kidney-Friendly Tuna Salad

Preparation Time: 10 min | Cooking Time: 0 min | Serving Size: 2 servings

Ingredients

- 1 can (5 ounces) low-sodium tuna, drained
- 1/4 cup diced celery
- 1/4 cup diced apple
- 2 tablespoons low-sodium mayonnaise
- 1 teaspoon lemon juice
- 1 tablespoon chopped fresh parsley
- Pepper to taste
- Lettuce leaves or whole wheat bread (low sodium) for serving

Step-by-Step Cooking Instructions

Combine Ingredients: In a bowl, mix the drained tuna, diced celery, diced apple, low-sodium mayonnaise, and lemon juice. Stir until well combined.

Add Flavor: Stir in the chopped parsley, and season with pepper to taste.

Chill (Optional): For best flavor, cover and refrigerate the tuna salad for about 30 minutes before serving.

Serve: Serve the tuna salad on a bed of lettuce leaves or spread between slices of low-sodium whole wheat bread for a satisfying sandwich.

Sodium: Approximately 150mg | Potassium: Approximately 200mg | Phosphorus: Approximately 150mg | Protein: Approximately 20g

This Kidney-Friendly Tuna Salad offers a refreshing and nutritious option for a light lunch or snack. Made with low-sodium ingredients and packed with protein, it's designed to fit well within a renal diet, supporting kidney health without sacrificing flavor. The addition of fresh apple and parsley not only adds a delightful crunch and freshness but also enhances the overall nutritional profile of the dish.

Asian-inspired Tofu and Sauteed Vegetables

Preparation Time: 15 min | Cooking Time: 20 min | Serving Size: 4 servings

Ingredients

- 1 block (14 ounces) firm tofu, pressed and cubed
- 2 tablespoons olive oil
- 1 cup broccoli florets
- 1/2 cup sliced carrots
- 1/2 cup bell pepper strips
- 1/2 cup snap peas
- 2 cloves garlic, minced
- 1 tablespoon grated ginger
- 1/4 cup low-sodium soy sauce or tamari
- 1 tablespoon rice vinegar
- 1 teaspoon sesame oil
- 1 tablespoon cornstarch dissolved in 2 tablespoons water (optional, for thickening)
- Sesame seeds for garnish

Step-by-Step Cooking Instructions

Prep Tofu: Press the tofu to remove excess moisture, then cut into 1-inch cubes.
Cook Tofu: Heat 1 tablespoon of olive oil in a large skillet or wok over medium-high heat. Add tofu cubes and cook until golden brown on all sides, about 10 minutes. Remove tofu and set aside.
Sauté Vegetables: In the same skillet, add the remaining tablespoon of olive oil. Add broccoli, carrots, bell pepper, snap peas, garlic, and ginger. Sauté until vegetables are tender-crisp, about 5-7 minutes.
Combine: Return the tofu to the skillet with the vegetables. In a small bowl, mix low-sodium soy sauce, rice vinegar, and sesame oil. Pour the sauce over the tofu and vegetables, stirring to combine. If desired, add the cornstarch mixture to thicken the sauce. Cook for an additional 2-3 minutes.
Garnish and Serve: Sprinkle with sesame seeds before serving.

Sodium: Approximately 200mg | Potassium: Approximately 300mg | Phosphorus: Approximately 150mg | Protein: Approximately 12g

Pasta Primavera with Garlic Olive Oil Sauce

Preparation Time: 10 min | Cooking Time: 20 min | Serving Size: 4 servings

Ingredients

- 8 oz whole wheat pasta
- 2 tablespoons olive oil
- 3 cloves garlic, minced
- 1 cup broccoli florets
- 1/2 cup sliced carrots
- 1/2 cup cherry tomatoes, halved
- 1/2 cup sliced bell peppers
- 1/4 cup peas
- Salt (optional) and pepper to taste
- Fresh basil leaves for garnish

Step-by-Step Cooking Instructions

Cook Pasta: Bring a large pot of water to a boil. Add the pasta and cook according to package instructions until al dente. Drain and set aside.
Sauté Garlic: In a large skillet, heat the olive oil over medium heat. Add the minced garlic and sauté for about 1 minute, or until fragrant.
Add Vegetables: To the skillet, add broccoli, carrots, cherry tomatoes, bell peppers, and peas. Sauté for about 5-7 minutes, or until the vegetables are tender yet crisp.
Combine Pasta and Vegetables: Add the cooked pasta to the skillet with the vegetables. Toss well to combine. Season with salt (optional) and pepper to taste.
Serve: Divide the pasta among plates. Garnish with fresh basil leaves before serving.

Sodium: Approximately 50mg | Potassium: Approximately 200mg | Phosphorus: Approximately 100mg | Protein: Approximately 8g

This Pasta Primavera with Garlic Olive Oil Sauce is a fresh and flavorful dish perfect for those following a renal diet. Made with whole wheat pasta and a variety of colorful vegetables, it's a nutritious meal that's low in sodium, potassium, and phosphorus. The garlic olive oil sauce adds a simple yet delicious coating to the pasta and vegetables, making it a delightful choice for a kidney-friendly diet.

Roasted Beet and Goat Cheese Salad

Preparation Time: 15 min | Cooking Time: 45 min | Serving Size: 4 servings

Ingredients

- 4 medium beets, cleaned and trimmed
- 2 tablespoons olive oil
- 1/2 cup goat cheese, crumbled
- 2 cups mixed salad greens
- 1/4 cup walnuts, chopped
- 2 tablespoons balsamic vinegar
- Salt (optional) and pepper to taste

Step-by-Step Cooking Instructions

Roast Beets: Preheat the oven to 400°F (200°C). Toss the beets with 1 tablespoon olive oil and wrap them individually in foil. Roast in the preheated oven until tender, about 45 minutes. Once cool, peel and slice.

Prepare Salad: In a large bowl, combine the mixed salad greens, sliced roasted beets, crumbled goat cheese, and chopped walnuts.

Dressing: In a small bowl, whisk together the remaining olive oil and balsamic vinegar. Season with salt (optional) and pepper.

Combine: Drizzle the dressing over the salad and gently toss to coat.

Serve: Divide the salad among plates and serve immediately.

Sodium: Approximately 130mg | Potassium: Approximately 400mg | Phosphorus: Approximately 120mg | Protein: Approximately 7g

This Roasted Beet and Goat Cheese Salad is a colorful and nutritious option, perfect for those managing their kidney health. The combination of earthy beets, creamy goat cheese, crunchy walnuts, and tangy balsamic dressing creates a delightful variety of textures and flavors. This dish is not only delicious but also kidney-friendly, with careful consideration given to the sodium, potassium, phosphorus, and protein content to fit within a renal diet.

Chicken and Rice Soup

Preparation Time: 10 min | Cooking Time: 30 min | Serving Size: 4 servings

Ingredients

- 2 tablespoons olive oil
- 1 small onion, diced
- 2 carrots, peeled and diced
- 2 celery stalks, diced
- 2 cloves garlic, minced
- 6 cups low-sodium chicken broth
- 1 cup cooked white rice
- 2 cups cooked, shredded chicken breast
- Salt (optional) and pepper to taste
- 2 tablespoons fresh parsley, chopped

Step-by-Step Cooking Instructions

Sauté Vegetables: In a large pot, heat the olive oil over medium heat. Add the onion, carrots, celery, and garlic. Sauté until the vegetables are soft, about 5 minutes.
Add Broth: Pour in the low-sodium chicken broth and bring to a simmer.
Add Chicken and Rice: Stir in the cooked white rice and shredded chicken breast. Season with salt (optional) and pepper. Simmer for 20 minutes, allowing the flavors to meld.
Finish and Serve: Stir in the fresh parsley just before serving. Ladle the soup into bowls.

Sodium: Approximately 150mg | Potassium: Approximately 250mg | Phosphorus: Approximately 120mg | Protein: Approximately 20g

This Chicken and Rice Soup is a comforting and nourishing meal, perfect for those on a renal diet. It's packed with wholesome ingredients and provides a good balance of nutrients while keeping sodium, potassium, and phosphorus levels in check. Enjoy this warming soup any time you need a simple and satisfying meal.

Avocado Chicken Salad

Preparation Time: 15 min | Cooking Time: 0 min | Serving Size: 4 servings

Ingredients

- 2 cups cooked and shredded chicken breast
- 1 ripe avocado, diced
- 1/2 cup cherry tomatoes, halved
- 1/4 cup red onion, finely chopped
- 2 tablespoons cilantro, chopped
- Juice of 1 lime
- Salt (optional) and pepper to taste
- Lettuce leaves for serving

Step-by-Step Cooking Instructions

Combine Ingredients: In a large bowl, combine the shredded chicken, diced avocado, cherry tomatoes, red onion, and cilantro.

Dress the Salad: Add the lime juice to the salad and gently toss to coat all the ingredients. Season with salt (optional) and pepper to taste.

Chill: Let the salad chill in the refrigerator for about 10 minutes before serving to enhance the flavors.

Serve: Serve the avocado chicken salad on a bed of lettuce leaves.

Sodium: Approximately 70mg | Potassium: Approximately 400mg | Phosphorus: Approximately 200mg | Protein: Approximately 25g

Carrot Ginger Soup

Preparation Time: 10 min | Cooking Time: 30 min | Serving Size: 4 servings

Ingredients

- 1 tablespoon olive oil
- 1 onion, diced
- 2 cloves garlic, minced
- 2 tablespoons fresh ginger, grated
- 1 pound carrots, peeled and diced
- 4 cups low-sodium vegetable broth
- Salt (optional) and pepper to taste
- Fresh parsley for garnish

Step-by-Step Cooking Instructions

Sauté Aromatics: In a large pot, heat the olive oil over medium heat. Add the onion, garlic, and ginger, sautéing until the onion is translucent, about 5 minutes.

Cook Carrots: Add the diced carrots to the pot, stirring to combine with the aromatics. Cook for an additional 5 minutes.

Add Broth: Pour in the low-sodium vegetable broth. Bring the mixture to a boil, then reduce the heat and simmer, covered, until the carrots are tender, about 20 minutes.

Blend Soup: Use an immersion blender to puree the soup until smooth. Alternatively, carefully transfer the soup to a blender to puree in batches. Season with salt (optional) and pepper to taste.

Serve: Ladle the soup into bowls and garnish with fresh parsley before serving.

Sodium: Approximately 200mg | Potassium: Approximately 350mg | Phosphorus: Approximately 100mg | Protein: Approximately 2g

This Carrot Ginger Soup is a warming and nutritious choice, perfect for those following a renal diet. The combination of sweet carrots and spicy ginger creates a delightful flavor, while the use of low-sodium vegetable broth makes it suitable for managing sodium intake. This soup is not only easy to prepare but also offers the benefits of being low in potassium, phosphorus, and high in vitamins, making it a comforting and healthful meal option.

Spinach and Goat Cheese Stuffed Chicken Breast

Preparation Time: 20 min | Cooking Time: 25 min | Serving Size: 4 servings

Ingredients

- 4 boneless, skinless chicken breasts
- 1 cup fresh spinach, chopped
- 4 ounces goat cheese
- 2 cloves garlic, minced
- 1 tablespoon olive oil
- Salt (optional) and pepper to taste
- Toothpicks or kitchen twine for securing

Step-by-Step Cooking Instructions

Preheat Oven: Preheat your oven to 375°F (190°C).

Prepare Chicken: Slice each chicken breast horizontally to create a pocket, being careful not to cut all the way through.

Mix Filling: In a bowl, combine the chopped spinach, goat cheese, and minced garlic. Season with a bit of pepper.

Stuff Chicken: Evenly divide the spinach and goat cheese mixture among the chicken breasts, stuffing each pocket. Use toothpicks or kitchen twine to secure them closed.

Cook: Heat olive oil in a large oven-proof skillet over medium heat. Season the outside of the chicken breasts with salt (optional) and pepper. Sear each side of the chicken for about 3 minutes until golden brown.

Bake: Transfer the skillet to the oven and bake for 20 minutes, or until the chicken is cooked through and no longer pink in the center.

Serve: Let the chicken rest for a few minutes before serving. Remove toothpicks or twine before serving.

Sodium: Approximately 200mg | Potassium: Approximately 300mg | Phosphorus: Approximately 250mg | Protein: Approximately 30g

Cucumber Tomato Salad with Feta

Preparation Time: 10 min | Cooking Time: 0 min | Serving Size: 4 servings

Ingredients

- 2 large cucumbers, peeled and diced
- 2 large tomatoes, diced
- 1/2 red onion, thinly sliced
- 1/4 cup crumbled feta cheese (low sodium)
- 2 tablespoons olive oil
- 1 tablespoon vinegar (either red wine or apple cider)
- Salt (optional) and pepper to taste
- Fresh herbs (such as dill or parsley), chopped, for garnish

Step-by-Step Cooking Instructions

Combine Vegetables: In a large bowl, mix together the diced cucumbers, tomatoes, and sliced red onion.

Add Cheese and Dressing: Sprinkle the crumbled feta cheese over the vegetables. Drizzle with olive oil and vinegar. Gently toss to combine.

Season: Season with salt (optional) and pepper to taste.

Garnish and Serve: Garnish with fresh herbs before serving. Serve immediately or chill in the refrigerator for about 30 minutes to allow flavors to meld.

Sodium: Approximately 100mg | Potassium: Approximately 250mg | Phosphorus: Approximately 75mg | Protein: Approximately 4g

Roasted Turkey and Cranberry Wrap

Preparation Time: 15 min | Cooking Time: 0 min | Serving Size: 2 wraps

Ingredients

- 2 whole wheat tortillas (low sodium)
- 4 slices of low-sodium roasted turkey breast
- 2 tablespoons cranberry sauce (low sugar)
- 1/4 cup mixed greens or spinach
- 1/4 cup thinly sliced cucumber
- 1/4 avocado, thinly sliced
- Salt (optional) and pepper to taste

Step-by-Step Cooking Instructions

Prepare Ingredients: Lay out the whole wheat tortillas on a clean surface. Evenly spread 1 tablespoon of cranberry sauce on each tortilla.

Assemble Wraps: On one half of each tortilla, layer two slices of roasted turkey breast, a handful of mixed greens or spinach, cucumber slices, and avocado slices. Season with salt (optional) and pepper to taste.

Roll the Wraps: Carefully roll each tortilla tightly, starting from the side with the fillings, to enclose the contents. If necessary, use toothpicks to secure the wraps.

Serve: Cut each wrap in half, if desired, and serve immediately.

Sodium: Approximately 200mg | Potassium: Approximately 300mg | Phosphorus: Approximately 100mg | Protein: Approximately 15g

This Roasted Turkey and Cranberry Wrap combines the classic flavors of turkey and cranberry in a healthy, kidney-friendly package. The use of whole wheat tortillas adds fiber, while low-sodium turkey breast helps manage sodium intake. Cranberry sauce provides a touch of sweetness without adding too much sugar, making this wrap a balanced option for a renal diet. Fresh vegetables add crunch and nutritional value, rounding out this delicious and wholesome meal.

Caprese Salad with Balsamic Glaze

Preparation Time: 10 min | Cooking Time: 0 min | Serving Size: 4 servings

Ingredients

- 4 large ripe tomatoes, sliced
- 8 ounces fresh mozzarella cheese, sliced
- 1/4 cup fresh basil leaves
- 2 tablespoons balsamic glaze (low sodium)
- 2 tablespoons extra virgin olive oil
- Salt (optional) and pepper to taste

Step-by-Step Cooking Instructions

Arrange Salad: On a large platter, alternate layers of tomato slices, mozzarella cheese slices, and basil leaves.

Season: Drizzle the extra virgin olive oil evenly over the salad. Then, drizzle the balsamic glaze. Season with salt (optional) and pepper to taste.

Serve: Let the salad sit for about 5 minutes to allow flavors to meld before serving.

Sodium: Approximately 100mg | Potassium: Approximately 200mg | Phosphorus: Approximately 150mg | Protein: Approximately 8g

This Caprese Salad with Balsamic Glaze is a simple yet elegant dish perfect for those following a renal diet. The combination of fresh tomatoes, mozzarella, and basil with the richness of balsamic glaze and olive oil creates a timeless salad that's as nutritious as it is delicious. By choosing low-sodium ingredients, this version remains kidney-friendly while delivering classic Italian flavors.

Lentil Soup with Carrots and Celery

Preparation Time: 15 min | Cooking Time: 45 min | Serving Size: 6 servings

Ingredients

- 1 cup dried lentils, rinsed
- 2 tablespoons olive oil
- 1 large onion, diced
- 2 carrots, peeled and diced
- 2 stalks celery, diced
- 2 cloves garlic, minced
- 6 cups low-sodium vegetable broth
- 1 teaspoon dried thyme
- 1 bay leaf
- Salt (optional) and pepper to taste
- Fresh parsley, chopped, for garnish

Step-by-Step Cooking Instructions

Sauté Vegetables: In a large pot, heat the olive oil over medium heat. Add the onion, carrots, celery, and garlic. Sauté until the vegetables are softened, about 5 minutes.
Add Lentils and Broth: Stir in the lentils, low-sodium vegetable broth, dried thyme, and bay leaf. Bring to a boil, then reduce the heat and simmer, covered, for about 35-40 minutes, or until the lentils are tender.
Season: Remove the bay leaf. Season the soup with salt (optional) and pepper to taste.
Serve: Ladle the soup into bowls and garnish with fresh parsley.

Sodium: Approximately 100mg | Potassium: Approximately 365mg | Phosphorus: Approximately 200mg | Protein: Approximately 12g

Balsamic Grilled Vegetables

Preparation Time: 15 min | Cooking Time: 20 min | Serving Size: 4 servings

Ingredients

- 1 zucchini, sliced into rounds
- 1 yellow squash, sliced into rounds
- 1 red bell pepper, cut into strips
- 1 yellow bell pepper, cut into strips
- 1 red onion, cut into wedges
- 2 tablespoons olive oil
- 3 tablespoons balsamic vinegar
- Salt (optional) and pepper to taste
- 1 teaspoon dried Italian herbs

Step-by-Step Cooking Instructions

Prep Vegetables: Wash and slice all vegetables as described. Place them in a large bowl.

Season: Add olive oil, balsamic vinegar, salt (optional), pepper, and dried Italian herbs to the vegetables. Toss until well coated.

Grill: Preheat the grill to medium-high heat. Place vegetables in a grill basket or directly on the grill rack. Grill for about 10 minutes on each side or until vegetables are tender and have grill marks.

Serve: Remove the vegetables from the grill and serve immediately.

Sodium: Approximately 50mg | Potassium: Approximately 400mg | Phosphorus: Approximately 100mg | Protein: Approximately 2g

These Balsamic Grilled Vegetables are a colorful and healthy side dish perfect for any meal. The combination of zucchini, squash, bell peppers, and red onion, all marinated in a savory balsamic and herb mix, provides a delicious way to enjoy your veggies. Grilling enhances their natural flavors, while keeping the dish light and renal-diet friendly.

Quiche with Egg Whites and Vegetables

Preparation Time: 15 min | Cooking Time: 35 min | Serving Size: 6 servings

Ingredients

- 1 pre-made pie crust (low sodium)
- 1 cup egg whites
- 1/2 cup low-fat milk
- 1 cup spinach, chopped
- 1/2 cup mushrooms, sliced
- 1/2 cup red bell pepper, diced
- 1/4 cup onion, diced
- 1/2 cup low-sodium cheese, grated
- Salt (optional) and pepper to taste

Step-by-Step Cooking Instructions

Preheat Oven: Preheat your oven to 375°F (190°C).

Prepare Crust: Place the pre-made pie crust in a 9-inch pie pan. Pre-bake the crust for 8 minutes. Remove from oven.

Sauté Vegetables: In a skillet over medium heat, sauté the spinach, mushrooms, bell pepper, and onion until just tender, about 5 minutes. Season with salt (optional) and pepper.

Mix Eggs: In a bowl, whisk together the egg whites and milk until well combined. Stir in the sautéed vegetables and grated cheese.

Assemble Quiche: Pour the egg and vegetable mixture into the pre-baked crust.

Bake: Bake in the preheated oven for 25-30 minutes, or until the center is set and the top is lightly golden.

Serve: Let the quiche cool for a few minutes before slicing and serving.

Sodium: Approximately 150mg | Potassium: Approximately 200mg | Phosphorus: Approximately 100mg | Protein: Approximately 10g

Tabbouleh with Quinoa

Preparation Time: 15 min | Cooking Time: 15 min | Serving Size: 4 servings

Ingredients

- 1 cup quinoa
- 2 cups water
- 1 cup fresh parsley, finely chopped
- 1/2 cup fresh mint, finely chopped
- 1/2 cup tomato, diced
- 1/4 cup cucumber, diced
- 1/4 cup lemon juice
- 2 tablespoons olive oil
- Salt (optional) and pepper to taste

Step-by-Step Cooking Instructions

Cook Quinoa: Rinse quinoa under cold water. In a saucepan, bring 2 cups of water to a boil. Add quinoa, reduce heat to low, cover, and simmer for about 15 minutes, or until water is absorbed. Fluff with a fork and let cool.

Prepare Vegetables: While the quinoa is cooling, finely chop the parsley and mint, and dice the tomato and cucumber.

Combine: In a large bowl, mix the cooled quinoa with the chopped parsley, mint, tomato, and cucumber.

Dress the Salad: Add lemon juice and olive oil to the quinoa mixture. Season with salt (optional) and pepper to taste. Toss well to combine.

Chill and Serve: For best flavor, let the tabbouleh chill in the refrigerator for at least 30 minutes before serving.

Sodium: Approximately 10mg | Potassium: Approximately 250mg | Phosphorus: Approximately 150mg | Protein: Approximately 5g

Dinner Recipes

Dinner plays a crucial role in a renal diet, serving as the final meal of the day and a vital opportunity to ensure balanced nutrition that supports kidney health through the night. It's a time when individuals can reflect on their daily intake and adjust their meal to meet any remaining nutritional needs or restrictions. The goal of dinner within a renal diet is to provide a satisfying meal that maintains the balance of nutrients essential for kidney health, such as controlling sodium, potassium, phosphorus, and protein levels, without overburdening the kidneys before bedtime.

For those managing kidney health, dinner should be thoughtfully planned to include kidney-friendly foods that are rich in essential nutrients yet low in minerals that need to be limited, depending on individual health goals and kidney function. It's important to include high-quality protein sources that are easy on the kidneys, alongside a variety of vegetables and whole grains that contribute fiber, vitamins, and minerals to the diet.

Portion control is also a key factor in a renal diet, especially at dinner time, to avoid overconsumption of certain nutrients that could potentially stress the kidneys. Including a moderate portion of protein, a serving of whole grains or a starchy vegetable, and plenty of non-starchy vegetables can help create a balanced plate that supports kidney health and overall well-being.

Hydration is another aspect to consider at dinner, with a focus on consuming enough fluids throughout the day but being mindful not to overload the kidneys in the evening. Opting for low-potassium beverages or simply water can aid in hydration without contributing excess potassium to the diet.

The dinner recipes in this section are designed with these principles in mind, offering delicious and nutritious options that cater to the needs of those on a renal diet. Each recipe aims to deliver balanced nutrition that satisfies taste buds while keeping kidney health at the forefront, ensuring a peaceful and supportive rest through the night.

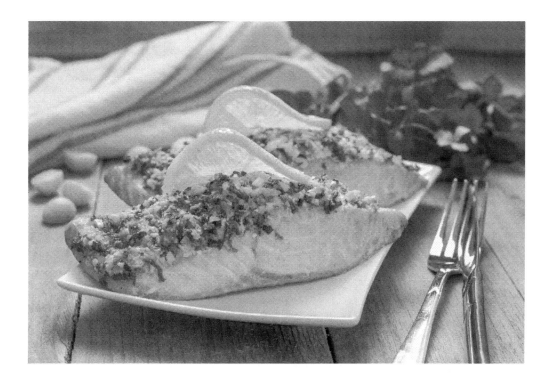

Baked Salmon with Herb Crust

Preparation Time: 10 min | Cooking Time: 20 min | Serving Size: 4 servings

Ingredients

- 4 salmon fillets (about 6 ounces each)
- 2 tablespoons olive oil
- 1/4 cup fresh parsley, finely chopped
- 1/4 cup fresh dill, finely chopped
- 2 cloves garlic, minced
- 1 teaspoon lemon zest
- Salt (optional) and pepper to taste
- Lemon wedges for serving

Step-by-Step Cooking Instructions

Preheat Oven: Preheat your oven to 400°F (200°C). Line a baking sheet with parchment paper.

Prepare Herb Mixture: In a small bowl, combine the olive oil, chopped parsley, dill, minced garlic, and lemon zest. Season with salt (optional) and pepper.

Season Salmon: Place the salmon fillets on the prepared baking sheet. Brush each fillet with the herb mixture, ensuring they are well coated.

Bake: Place the salmon in the preheated oven and bake for about 15-20 minutes, or until the salmon flakes easily with a fork.

Serve: Serve the salmon immediately, garnished with lemon wedges.

Sodium: Approximately 75mg | Potassium: Approximately 500mg | Phosphorus: Approximately 250mg | Protein: Approximately 23g

This Baked Salmon with Herb Crust is a flavorful and kidney-friendly dish perfect for a nourishing dinner. The combination of fresh herbs and lemon zest creates a vibrant crust that complements the rich, fatty profile of the salmon, offering a delicious way to enjoy essential nutrients beneficial for kidney health. Low in sodium and phosphorus while being a great source of high-quality protein, this dish supports the dietary needs of those managing kidney health, ensuring a delicious end to the day that doesn't compromise on nutritional requirements.

Stir-Fried Beef and Broccoli

Preparation Time: 15 min | Cooking Time: 10 min | Serving Size: 4 servings

Ingredients

- 1 pound lean beef (such as flank steak), thinly sliced
- 4 cups broccoli florets
- 2 tablespoons olive oil
- 1/4 cup low-sodium soy sauce or tamari
- 1 tablespoon cornstarch
- 2 cloves garlic, minced
- 1 teaspoon ginger, minced
- 1/2 cup water
- Pepper to taste

Step-by-Step Cooking Instructions

Marinate Beef: In a bowl, mix the cornstarch and low-sodium soy sauce. Add the thinly sliced beef, ensuring each piece is coated. Let it marinate for at least 10 minutes.

Prepare Vegetables: Steam the broccoli florets until they are just tender, about 3-4 minutes. Set aside.

Cook Beef: Heat 1 tablespoon of olive oil in a large skillet or wok over medium-high heat. Add the beef slices in a single layer, working in batches if necessary, and stir-fry until browned. Remove beef and set aside.

Sauté Garlic and Ginger: Add the remaining tablespoon of olive oil to the skillet. Sauté the minced garlic and ginger for about 1 minute, or until fragrant.

Combine Ingredients: Return the beef to the skillet with the garlic and ginger. Add the steamed broccoli and water. Stir well and cook for an additional 2-3 minutes, allowing the sauce to thicken slightly.

Season and Serve: Season with pepper to taste. Serve hot.

Sodium: Approximately 300mg | Potassium: Approximately 400mg | Phosphorus: Approximately 250mg | Protein: Approximately 25g

Vegetarian Chili

Preparation Time: 15 min | Cooking Time: 30 min | Serving Size: 6 servings

Ingredients

- 1 tablespoon olive oil
- 1 large onion, chopped
- 2 cloves garlic, minced
- 2 bell peppers (any color), diced
- 2 carrots, peeled and diced
- 1 zucchini, diced
- 1 cup low-sodium canned kidney beans, rinsed and drained
- 1 cup low-sodium canned black beans, rinsed and drained
- 2 cups low-sodium tomato sauce
- 1 cup water
- 2 teaspoons chili powder
- 1 teaspoon cumin
- Salt (optional) and pepper to taste
- Fresh cilantro for garnish

-

Step-by-Step Cooking Instructions

Sauté Vegetables: In a large pot, heat the olive oil over medium heat. Add the onion and garlic, sautéing until soft. Add the bell peppers, carrots, and zucchini, cooking until they start to soften, about 5 minutes.

Add Beans and Seasonings: Stir in the kidney beans, black beans, tomato sauce, water, chili powder, and cumin. Season with salt (optional) and pepper. Bring to a simmer.

Simmer: Reduce heat to low and let the chili simmer, covered, for about 25 minutes, stirring occasionally.

Garnish and Serve: Serve the chili hot, garnished with fresh cilantro.

Sodium: Approximately 200mg | Potassium: Approximately 400mg | Phosphorus: Approximately 150mg | Protein: Approximately 8g

Lemon Garlic Halibut

Preparation Time: 10 min | Cooking Time: 15 min | Serving Size: 4 servings

Ingredients

- 4 halibut fillets (6 ounces each)
- 2 tablespoons olive oil
- 4 cloves garlic, minced
- Juice of 1 lemon
- Zest of 1 lemon
- Salt (optional) and pepper to taste
- Fresh parsley, chopped, for garnish

Step-by-Step Cooking Instructions

Preheat Oven: Preheat your oven to 375°F (190°C).

Prepare Garlic Lemon Sauce: In a small bowl, mix together the olive oil, minced garlic, lemon juice, and lemon zest. Season with salt (optional) and pepper.

Season Halibut: Place the halibut fillets in a baking dish. Spoon the garlic lemon sauce over the fillets, ensuring they are evenly coated.

Bake: Place the baking dish in the preheated oven and bake for about 12-15 minutes, or until the halibut flakes easily with a fork.

Garnish and Serve: Remove from oven and garnish with fresh parsley. Serve immediately.

Sodium: Approximately 70mg | Potassium: Approximately 500mg | Phosphorus: Approximately 250mg | Protein: Approximately 22g

Beef Stir-Fry with Broccoli and Bell Peppers

Preparation Time: 15 min | Cooking Time: 10 min | Serving Size: 4 servings

Ingredients

- 1 pound lean beef, thinly sliced (such as flank steak)
- 2 cups broccoli florets
- 1 red bell pepper, thinly sliced
- 1 yellow bell pepper, thinly sliced
- 2 tablespoons olive oil
- 1/4 cup low-sodium soy sauce
- 1 tablespoon ginger, minced
- 2 cloves garlic, minced
- 1 tablespoon cornstarch mixed with 2 tablespoons water
- Salt (optional) and pepper to taste

Step-by-Step Cooking Instructions

Marinate Beef: In a bowl, combine the beef with the low-sodium soy sauce, ginger, and garlic. Let it marinate for at least 10 minutes.

Cook Beef: Heat 1 tablespoon olive oil in a large skillet or wok over medium-high heat. Add the marinated beef and stir-fry until browned and cooked through, about 3-4 minutes. Remove beef from the skillet and set aside.

Sauté Vegetables: In the same skillet, add the remaining tablespoon of olive oil. Add the broccoli and bell peppers, stir-frying until they are vibrant and tender-crisp, about 3-5 minutes.

Thicken Sauce: Return the beef to the skillet with the vegetables. Stir the cornstarch and water mixture into the skillet. Cook, stirring constantly, until the sauce has thickened, about 1-2 minutes.

Season and Serve: Season with salt (optional) and pepper to taste. Serve immediately.

Sodium: Approximately 200mg | Potassium: Approximately 500mg | Phosphorus: Approximately 250mg | Protein: Approximately 26g

Baked Salmon with Dill

Preparation Time: 10 min | Cooking Time: 15 min | Serving Size: 4 servings

Ingredients

- 4 salmon fillets (6 ounces each)
- 2 tablespoons olive oil
- 2 tablespoons fresh dill, chopped
- Juice of 1 lemon
- Salt (optional) and pepper to taste
- Lemon slices for garnish

Step-by-Step Cooking Instructions

Preheat Oven: Preheat your oven to 400°F (200°C). Line a baking sheet with parchment paper.

Prepare Salmon: Place the salmon fillets on the prepared baking sheet. Brush each fillet with olive oil. Sprinkle with chopped dill, and drizzle with lemon juice. Season with salt (optional) and pepper.

Bake: Bake in the preheated oven for about 12-15 minutes, or until the salmon flakes easily with a fork.

Serve: Garnish with lemon slices and serve immediately.

Sodium: Approximately 50mg | Potassium: Approximately 500mg | Phosphorus: Approximately 250mg | Protein: Approximately 23g

Vegetarian Chili

Preparation Time: 15 min | Cooking Time: 30 min | Serving Size: 6 servings

Ingredients

- 1 tablespoon olive oil
- 1 large onion, chopped
- 2 cloves garlic, minced
- 2 bell peppers (any color), diced
- 2 carrots, peeled and diced
- 2 zucchinis, diced
- 1 cup low-sodium canned kidney beans, rinsed and drained
- 1 cup low-sodium canned black beans, rinsed and drained
- 2 cups low-sodium tomato sauce
- 1 cup water
- 2 teaspoons chili powder
- 1 teaspoon cumin
- Salt (optional) and pepper to taste
- Fresh cilantro for garnish

Step-by-Step Cooking Instructions

Sauté Vegetables: In a large pot, heat the olive oil over medium heat. Add the onion and garlic, sautéing until soft. Add the bell peppers, carrots, and zucchini, cooking until they start to soften, about 5 minutes.

Add Beans and Seasonings: Stir in the kidney beans, black beans, tomato sauce, water, chili powder, and cumin. Season with salt (optional) and pepper. Bring to a simmer.

Simmer: Reduce heat to low and let the chili simmer, covered, for about 25 minutes, stirring occasionally.

Garnish and Serve: Serve the chili hot, garnished with fresh cilantro.

Sodium: Approximately 200mg | Potassium: Approximately 400mg | Phosphorus: Approximately 150mg | Protein: Approximately 8g

Roast Chicken with Herbs

Preparation Time: 20 min | Cooking Time: 1 hr 30 min | Serving Size: 6 servings

Ingredients

- 1 whole chicken (about 4-5 pounds)
- 2 tablespoons olive oil
- 1 tablespoon fresh rosemary, chopped
- 1 tablespoon fresh thyme, chopped
- 1 tablespoon fresh parsley, chopped
- 2 cloves garlic, minced
- Salt (optional) and pepper to taste
- 1 lemon, halved

Step-by-Step Cooking Instructions

Preheat Oven: Preheat your oven to 375°F (190°C).

Prepare Chicken: Rinse the chicken and pat dry with paper towels. Rub the outside and inside of the chicken with olive oil.

Season: Mix the chopped herbs and minced garlic together. Season the chicken with this herb mixture, salt (optional), and pepper, both outside and in the cavity. Place the lemon halves inside the chicken cavity.

Roast: Place the chicken in a roasting pan, breast side up. Roast in the preheated oven for about 1 hour and 30 minutes, or until the internal temperature reaches 165°F (74°C) and the juices run clear.

Rest and Serve: Let the chicken rest for 10 minutes before carving. Serve with your choice of sides.

Sodium: Approximately 70mg | Potassium: Approximately 300mg | Phosphorus: Approximately 250mg | Protein: Approximately 25g

Spaghetti with Olive Oil and Garlic

Preparation Time: 5 min | Cooking Time: 15 min | Serving Size: 4 servings

Ingredients

- 8 ounces spaghetti (whole wheat, if preferred)
- 1/4 cup olive oil
- 4 cloves garlic, thinly sliced
- Red pepper flakes (optional, to taste)
- Salt (optional) and pepper to taste
- Fresh parsley, chopped, for garnish
- Grated Parmesan cheese (optional, low sodium), for serving

Step-by-Step Cooking Instructions

Cook Spaghetti: Bring a large pot of water to a boil. Add the spaghetti and cook according to package instructions until al dente. Drain, reserving 1 cup of pasta water.

Sauté Garlic: While the pasta cooks, heat the olive oil in a large skillet over medium heat. Add the garlic slices and red pepper flakes (if using). Sauté until the garlic is golden brown, about 2 minutes. Be careful not to burn the garlic.

Combine: Add the drained spaghetti to the skillet with the garlic and olive oil. Toss well to coat. If the pasta seems dry, add a little of the reserved pasta water until it reaches your desired consistency.

Season: Season with salt (optional) and pepper to taste.

Serve: Garnish with chopped parsley and grated Parmesan cheese (if using). Serve immediately.

Sodium: Approximately 30mg (without added salt) | Potassium: Approximately 150mg | Phosphorus: Approximately 100mg | Protein: Approximately 8g

Grilled Pork Chops with Apple Slaw

Preparation Time: 20 min | Cooking Time: 15 min | Serving Size: 4 servings

Ingredients

- 4 boneless pork chops, about 1-inch thick
- 2 tablespoons olive oil
- Salt (optional) and pepper to taste
- **For the Apple Slaw:**
    - 2 medium apples, julienned
    - 1/4 cabbage, thinly sliced
    - 1 carrot, julienned
    - 2 tablespoons apple cider vinegar
    - 1 teaspoon honey
    - 1 tablespoon olive oil
    - Salt (optional) and pepper to taste

Step-by-Step Cooking Instructions

Preheat Grill: Preheat your grill to medium-high heat.
Season Pork Chops: Brush pork chops with olive oil and season with salt (optional) and pepper.
Grill Pork Chops: Grill the pork chops for about 7-8 minutes on each side, or until they reach an internal temperature of 145°F (63°C). Remove from the grill and let rest for 3 minutes.
Prepare Apple Slaw: In a large bowl, combine the julienned apples, sliced cabbage, julienned carrot, apple cider vinegar, honey, and olive oil. Toss until well mixed. Season with salt (optional) and pepper to taste.
Serve: Serve the grilled pork chops with a side of apple slaw.

Sodium: Approximately 70mg | Potassium: Approximately 500mg | Phosphorus: Approximately 250mg | Protein: Approximately 25g

Lemon Herb Baked Tilapia with Zucchini Ribbons

Preparation Time: 15 min | Cooking Time: 20 min | Serving Size: 4 servings

Ingredients

- 4 tilapia fillets (about 6 ounces each)
- 2 tablespoons olive oil
- 1 lemon, juiced and zested
- 2 teaspoons dried Italian herbs (basil, oregano, thyme)
- Salt (optional) and pepper to taste
- 2 medium zucchinis, cut into ribbons with a vegetable peeler
- 1 tablespoon fresh parsley, chopped (for garnish)

Step-by-Step Cooking Instructions

Preheat Oven: Preheat your oven to 400°F (200°C).

Season Tilapia: In a small bowl, combine olive oil, lemon juice and zest, Italian herbs, and optional salt and pepper. Brush both sides of the tilapia fillets with the mixture.

Prepare Baking Dish: Place the seasoned tilapia fillets in a baking dish. Surround them with zucchini ribbons.

Bake: Bake in the preheated oven for about 20 minutes, or until the fish flakes easily with a fork.

Garnish and Serve: Garnish the baked tilapia and zucchini ribbons with fresh parsley before serving.

Sodium: Approximately 60mg | Potassium: Approximately 550mg | Phosphorus: Approximately 200mg | Protein: Approximately 28g

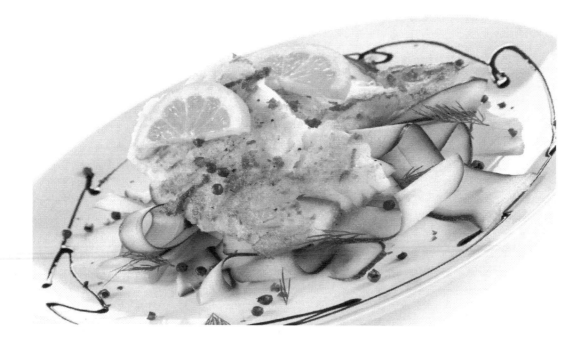

Ratatouille

Preparation Time: 25 min | Cooking Time: 40 min | Serving Size: 6 servings

Ingredients

- 1 eggplant, cut into ½-inch pieces
- 2 zucchinis, sliced into ½-inch rounds
- 2 yellow squashes, sliced into ½-inch rounds
- 1 red bell pepper, chopped
- 1 yellow bell pepper, chopped
- 2 tomatoes, chopped
- 1 onion, diced
- 3 cloves garlic, minced
- 2 tablespoons olive oil
- 1 teaspoon dried thyme
- 1 teaspoon dried oregano
- Salt (optional) and pepper to taste
- Fresh basil leaves, for garnish

Step-by-Step Cooking Instructions

Prepare Vegetables: Preheat the oven to 375°F (190°C). In a large mixing bowl, combine eggplant, zucchinis, yellow squashes, bell peppers, tomatoes, onion, and garlic. Drizzle with olive oil and season with thyme, oregano, optional salt, and pepper. Toss to coat evenly.

Bake: Transfer the vegetable mixture to a large baking dish. Spread out the vegetables evenly. Bake in the preheated oven for about 40 minutes, or until vegetables are tender and lightly browned.

Garnish and Serve: Garnish the ratatouille with fresh basil leaves before serving. This dish can be served hot or at room temperature.

Sodium: Approximately 30mg | Potassium: Approximately 650mg | Phosphorus: Approximately 120mg | Protein: Approximately 4g

Turkey Meatballs in Tomato Sauce

Preparation Time: 20 min | Cooking Time: 30 min | Serving Size: 4 servings

Ingredients

For the Meatballs:

- 1 pound ground turkey
- 1 egg, beaten
- 1/4 cup breadcrumbs
- 1/4 cup grated Parmesan cheese
- 1 teaspoon dried oregano
- 1 teaspoon dried basil
- Salt (optional) and pepper to taste

For the Tomato Sauce:

- 2 tablespoons olive oil
- 1 onion, finely chopped
- 2 cloves garlic, minced
- 1 can (28 ounces) no-salt-added crushed tomatoes
- 1 teaspoon dried oregano
- 1 teaspoon dried basil
- Salt (optional) and pepper to taste

Step-by-Step Cooking Instructions

Prepare Meatballs: In a bowl, mix together the ground turkey, egg, breadcrumbs, Parmesan cheese, oregano, basil, and optional salt and pepper. Form into 1-inch meatballs.

Brown Meatballs: In a large skillet over medium heat, add 1 tablespoon olive oil. Add the meatballs and cook until browned on all sides, about 5-7 minutes. Remove meatballs and set aside.

Make Tomato Sauce: In the same skillet, add the remaining olive oil. Add onion and garlic, and sauté until soft. Stir in crushed tomatoes, oregano, basil, and optional salt and pepper. Bring to a simmer.

Cook Meatballs in Sauce: Return the meatballs to the skillet, cover, and simmer for 20 minutes, or until the meatballs are cooked through.

Serve: Serve the turkey meatballs and tomato sauce hot, over cooked pasta, rice, or zucchini noodles if desired.

Sodium: Approximately 200mg | Potassium: Approximately 700mg | Phosphorus: Approximately 250mg | Protein: Approximately 27g

Baked Cod with Parsley Pesto

Preparation Time: 15 min | Cooking Time: 20 min | Serving Size: 4 servings

Ingredients

For the Cod:

- 4 cod fillets (about 6 ounces each)
- 2 tablespoons olive oil
- Salt (optional) and pepper to taste

For the Parsley Pesto:

- 1 cup fresh parsley leaves
- 1/4 cup almonds, toasted
- 2 cloves garlic
- 1/4 cup grated Parmesan cheese
- 1/2 cup olive oil
- Salt (optional) and pepper to taste

Step-by-Step Cooking Instructions

Preheat Oven: Preheat your oven to 400°F (200°C).

Prepare Cod: Place the cod fillets on a baking sheet. Brush each fillet with olive oil and season with optional salt and pepper.

Bake Cod: Bake in the preheated oven for about 15-20 minutes, or until the fish flakes easily with a fork.

Make Parsley Pesto: While the cod is baking, combine parsley, almonds, garlic, Parmesan cheese, and olive oil in a food processor. Blend until smooth. Season with optional salt and pepper to taste.

Serve: Serve the baked cod topped with a generous spoonful of parsley pesto.

Sodium: Approximately 120mg | Potassium: Approximately 500mg | Phosphorus: Approximately 250mg | Protein: Approximately 30g

Garlic Lemon Chicken Kebabs

Preparation Time: 15 min | Cooking Time: 10 min | Serving Size: 4 servings

Ingredients

- 1 pound chicken breast, cut into 1-inch pieces
- 2 tablespoons olive oil
- 2 cloves garlic, minced
- 1 lemon, zest and juice
- 1 teaspoon dried oregano
- Salt (optional) and pepper to taste
- 1 red bell pepper, cut into 1-inch pieces
- 1 yellow bell pepper, cut into 1-inch pieces
- 1 zucchini, sliced into ½-inch thick rounds
- 8 wooden or metal skewers (if using wooden skewers, soak in water for 30 minutes before using)

Step-by-Step Cooking Instructions

Marinate Chicken: In a large bowl, combine olive oil, minced garlic, lemon zest, lemon juice, oregano, and optional salt and pepper. Add chicken pieces and toss to coat. Cover and marinate in the refrigerator for at least 30 minutes, up to 2 hours.
Preheat Grill: Preheat your grill or grill pan to medium-high heat.
Assemble Kebabs: Thread the marinated chicken pieces alternately with red bell pepper, yellow bell pepper, and zucchini slices onto skewers.
Grill Kebabs: Grill the kebabs, turning occasionally, until the chicken is cooked through and vegetables are slightly charred, about 10 minutes.
Serve: Serve the kebabs hot, with additional lemon wedges on the side if desired.

Sodium: Approximately 85mg | Potassium: Approximately 600mg | Phosphorus: Approximately 300mg | Protein: Approximately 26g

Maple Glazed Salmon

Preparation Time: 10 min | Cooking Time: 15 min | Serving Size: 4 servings

Ingredients

- 4 salmon fillets (about 6 ounces each)
- 2 tablespoons maple syrup
- 1 tablespoon soy sauce (low sodium)
- 1 garlic clove, minced
- 1 teaspoon fresh ginger, grated
- Salt (optional) and pepper to taste
- 1 tablespoon olive oil

Step-by-Step Cooking Instructions

Preheat Oven: Preheat your oven to 400°F (200°C).

Prepare Glaze: In a small bowl, mix together the maple syrup, low sodium soy sauce, minced garlic, and grated ginger. Season with optional salt and pepper to taste.

Season Salmon: Place the salmon fillets on a baking tray lined with parchment paper. Brush each fillet with olive oil, then with the maple glaze.

Bake: Bake in the preheated oven for about 12-15 minutes, or until the salmon is cooked through and flakes easily with a fork.

Serve: Serve the maple glazed salmon hot, drizzling any remaining glaze from the tray over the fillets.

Sodium: Approximately 180mg | Potassium: Approximately 500mg | Phosphorus: Approximately 250mg | Protein: Approximately 23g

This Maple Glazed Salmon recipe offers a perfect balance of sweet and savory flavors, making it an enticing option for those managing their kidney health. The rich, omega-3 fatty acids in salmon are paired with the natural sweetness of maple syrup and the umami depth of low sodium soy sauce, creating a deliciously healthy dish. Designed with a renal diet in mind, this recipe keeps a close eye on sodium, potassium, phosphorus, and protein content, ensuring a nutritious meal without sacrificing taste.

Beef and Vegetable Kabobs

Preparation Time: 20 min | Cooking Time: 10 min | Serving Size: 4 servings

Ingredients

- 1 pound beef tenderloin, cut into 1-inch cubes
- 1 red bell pepper, cut into 1-inch pieces
- 1 yellow bell pepper, cut into 1-inch pieces
- 1 zucchini, sliced into ½-inch thick rounds
- 1 red onion, cut into wedges
- 2 tablespoons olive oil
- 1 teaspoon garlic powder
- 1 teaspoon dried rosemary
- Salt (optional) and pepper to taste
- 8 wooden or metal skewers (if using wooden skewers, soak in water for 30 minutes before using)

Step-by-Step Cooking Instructions

Marinate Beef: In a large bowl, combine beef cubes with olive oil, garlic powder, dried rosemary, and optional salt and pepper. Toss to coat evenly. Let marinate for at least 15 minutes, up to 2 hours in the refrigerator.

Preheat Grill: Preheat your grill or grill pan to medium-high heat.

Assemble Kabobs: Thread the marinated beef, bell peppers, zucchini, and red onion alternately onto skewers.

Grill Kabobs: Grill the kabobs, turning occasionally, until the beef is cooked to your liking and vegetables are slightly charred, about 10 minutes for medium-rare.

Serve: Serve the beef and vegetable kabobs hot, with side dishes of choice.

Sodium: Approximately 90mg | Potassium: Approximately 650mg | Phosphorus: Approximately 290mg | Protein: Approximately 26g

Vegetarian Stuffed Acorn Squash

Preparation Time: 15 min | Cooking Time: 45 min | Serving Size: 4 servings

Ingredients

- 2 acorn squashes, halved and seeded
- 1 tablespoon olive oil
- Salt (optional) and pepper to taste
- 1 cup quinoa, cooked
- 1/2 cup cranberries
- 1/2 cup pecans, chopped
- 1/2 cup feta cheese, crumbled
- 2 tablespoons maple syrup
- 1 teaspoon cinnamon
- 1/2 teaspoon nutmeg

Step-by-Step Cooking Instructions

Preheat Oven: Preheat your oven to 375°F (190°C).

Prepare Squash: Brush the inside of each acorn squash half with olive oil. Season with optional salt and pepper. Place squash halves cut-side down on a baking sheet.

Bake Squash: Bake in the preheated oven for about 25-30 minutes, or until the flesh is tender when pierced with a fork.

Mix Filling: In a bowl, combine cooked quinoa, cranberries, pecans, feta cheese, maple syrup, cinnamon, and nutmeg.

Stuff Squash: Once the squash halves are tender, remove from oven and flip them over. Fill each half with the quinoa mixture.

Bake Again: Return the stuffed squashes to the oven and bake for another 15 minutes.

Serve: Serve warm, drizzled with additional maple syrup if desired.

Sodium: Approximately 120mg | Potassium: Approximately 500mg | Phosphorus: Approximately 150mg | Protein: Approximately 6g

Chicken Piccata

Preparation Time: 15 min | Cooking Time: 20 min | Serving Size: 4 servings

Ingredients

- 4 boneless, skinless chicken breasts, pounded to even thickness
- 1/4 cup all-purpose flour (for dredging)
- 2 tablespoons olive oil
- Salt (optional) and pepper to taste
- 1/3 cup fresh lemon juice
- 1/2 cup low-sodium chicken broth
- 2 tablespoons capers, rinsed
- 2 tablespoons unsalted butter
- 2 tablespoons fresh parsley, chopped

Step-by-Step Cooking Instructions

Prepare Chicken: Season both sides of the chicken breasts with optional salt and pepper. Dredge in flour, shaking off any excess.

Cook Chicken: In a large skillet, heat olive oil over medium-high heat. Add chicken and cook until golden brown on both sides and cooked through, about 3-4 minutes per side. Remove chicken from the skillet and set aside.

Make Sauce: To the same skillet, add lemon juice, low-sodium chicken broth, and capers. Bring to a simmer, scraping up any browned bits from the bottom of the skillet. Stir in butter until melted and the sauce has slightly thickened.

Serve: Return the chicken to the skillet, spooning the sauce over the top. Simmer for an additional 2-3 minutes to reheat the chicken. Garnish with fresh parsley before serving.

Sodium: Approximately 125mg | Potassium: Approximately 300mg | Phosphorus: Approximately 220mg | Protein: Approximately 26g

Shrimp Scampi with Zoodles

Preparation Time: 20 min | Cooking Time: 10 min | Serving Size: 4 servings

Ingredients

- 1 pound large shrimp, peeled and deveined
- 4 medium zucchinis, spiralized into zoodles
- 2 tablespoons olive oil
- 3 cloves garlic, minced
- 1/2 cup low-sodium chicken broth
- 1 lemon, zest and juice
- Salt (optional) and pepper to taste
- 2 tablespoons unsalted butter
- 2 tablespoons fresh parsley, chopped
- 1/4 teaspoon red pepper flakes (optional)

Step-by-Step Cooking Instructions

Prepare Shrimp: Season the shrimp with optional salt and pepper.

Cook Shrimp: In a large skillet, heat 1 tablespoon olive oil over medium heat. Add shrimp and cook until pink and opaque, about 2-3 minutes per side. Remove shrimp and set aside.

Sauté Garlic: In the same skillet, add the remaining olive oil and minced garlic. Sauté for about 1 minute, until fragrant.

Add Broth and Lemon: Stir in the low-sodium chicken broth, lemon zest, and lemon juice. Bring to a simmer and let reduce slightly, about 2-3 minutes.

Combine Shrimp and Zoodles: Return the shrimp to the skillet, adding the zoodles. Toss to combine and cook for 2-3 minutes, just until the zoodles are tender.

Finish: Stir in unsalted butter, chopped parsley, and optional red pepper flakes until the butter is melted and the dish is well combined.

Serve: Serve the shrimp scampi over the zoodles, garnished with additional parsley if desired.

Sodium: Approximately 200mg | Potassium: Approximately 400mg | Phosphorus: Approximately 250mg | Protein: Approximately 24g

Moroccan Tagine with Vegetables

Preparation Time: 20 min | Cooking Time: 40 min | Serving Size: 6 servings

Ingredients

- 2 tablespoons olive oil
- 1 large onion, chopped
- 3 cloves garlic, minced
- 1 teaspoon ground cumin
- 1 teaspoon ground coriander
- 1/2 teaspoon ground cinnamon
- 1/2 teaspoon ground turmeric
- 1/4 teaspoon cayenne pepper (optional)
- 2 carrots, peeled and sliced
- 2 sweet potatoes, peeled and cubed
- 1 zucchini, sliced
- 1 bell pepper, chopped
- 1 can (15 ounces) no-salt-added diced tomatoes
- 1 can (15 ounces) chickpeas, rinsed and drained
- 1/2 cup low-sodium vegetable broth
- Salt (optional) and pepper to taste
- 2 tablespoons fresh cilantro, chopped
- 2 tablespoons fresh parsley, chopped

Step-by-Step Cooking Instructions

Sauté Aromatics: In a large pot or tagine, heat olive oil over medium heat. Add onion and garlic, cooking until softened. Stir in cumin, coriander, cinnamon, turmeric, and optional cayenne pepper, cooking for 1 minute until fragrant.

Add Vegetables: Add carrots, sweet potatoes, zucchini, and bell pepper to the pot, stirring to coat with the spices.

Simmer: Stir in the diced tomatoes with their juice, chickpeas, and vegetable broth. Bring to a simmer, then reduce heat to low, cover, and cook for 30-35 minutes, or until vegetables are tender.

Final Touches: Season with optional salt and pepper. Stir in chopped cilantro and parsley just before serving.

Serve: Serve the tagine hot, alongside couscous or rice if desired.

Sodium: Approximately 70mg | Potassium: Approximately 600mg | Phosphorus: Approximately 200mg | Protein: Approximately 6g

Baked Tilapia with Mango Salsa

Preparation Time: 15 min | Cooking Time: 20 min | Serving Size: 4 servings

Ingredients

For the Tilapia:

- 4 tilapia fillets (about 6 ounces each)
- 2 tablespoons olive oil
- Salt (optional) and pepper to taste

For the Mango Salsa:

- 1 ripe mango, diced
- 1/2 red bell pepper, diced
- 1/4 cup red onion, finely chopped
- 1 small jalapeño, seeded and minced (optional)
- 1/4 cup cilantro, chopped
- Juice of 1 lime
- Salt (optional) and pepper to taste

Step-by-Step Cooking Instructions

Preheat Oven: Preheat your oven to 375°F (190°C).
Prepare Tilapia: Brush each tilapia fillet with olive oil and season with optional salt and pepper. Place the fillets on a baking sheet lined with parchment paper.
Bake Tilapia: Bake in the preheated oven for about 15-20 minutes, or until the fish flakes easily with a fork.
Make Mango Salsa: While the tilapia is baking, combine diced mango, red bell pepper, red onion, jalapeño (if using), cilantro, and lime juice in a bowl. Season with optional salt and pepper to taste.
Serve: Serve the baked tilapia topped with the fresh mango salsa.

Sodium: Approximately 85mg | Potassium: Approximately 500mg | Phosphorus: Approximately 250mg | Protein: Approximately 23g

Pork Loin with Apple Compote

Preparation Time: 15 min | Cooking Time: 60 min | Serving Size: 6 servings

Ingredients

For the Pork Loin:

- 2 pounds pork loin
- 2 tablespoons olive oil
- 1 teaspoon dried thyme
- Salt (optional) and pepper to taste

For the Apple Compote:

- 4 apples, peeled, cored, and diced
- 1/4 cup water
- 2 tablespoons sugar
- 1/2 teaspoon cinnamon

Step-by-Step Cooking Instructions

Preheat Oven: Preheat your oven to 375°F (190°C).

Prepare Pork Loin: Rub the pork loin with olive oil and season with thyme, and optional salt and pepper. Place in a roasting pan.

Roast Pork Loin: Roast in the preheated oven for about 1 hour, or until the internal temperature reaches 145°F (63°C). Let it rest for 10 minutes before slicing.

Make Apple Compote: While the pork is roasting, combine diced apples, water, sugar, and cinnamon in a saucepan over medium heat. Cook until apples are soft and the mixture has thickened, about 15-20 minutes, stirring occasionally.

Serve: Slice the pork loin and serve topped with the warm apple compote.

Sodium: Approximately 65mg | Potassium: Approximately 400mg | Phosphorus: Approximately 250mg | Protein: Approximately 31g

Italian Beef Stew

Preparation Time: 20 min | Cooking Time: 2 hours | Serving Size: 6 servings

Ingredients

- 2 pounds beef chuck, cut into 1-inch cubes
- 1/4 cup flour (for dredging)
- 2 tablespoons olive oil
- 1 large onion, chopped
- 3 cloves garlic, minced
- 1 cup low-sodium beef broth
- 1 can (14.5 ounces) no-salt-added diced tomatoes
- 2 carrots, peeled and sliced
- 2 celery stalks, chopped
- 1 teaspoon dried oregano
- 1 teaspoon dried basil
- Salt (optional) and pepper to taste
- 1/2 cup fresh parsley, chopped

Step-by-Step Cooking Instructions

Dredge Beef: Lightly coat the beef cubes with flour, shaking off any excess.
Brown Beef: In a large pot, heat olive oil over medium-high heat. Add beef in batches, browning on all sides. Remove browned beef and set aside.
Sauté Vegetables: In the same pot, add more oil if needed and sauté the onion and garlic until soft.
Cook Stew: Return the beef to the pot along with low-sodium beef broth, diced tomatoes with their juice, carrots, celery, oregano, and basil. Season with optional salt and pepper. Bring to a boil, then reduce heat to low, cover, and simmer for about 2 hours, or until the beef is tender.
Finish with Parsley: Stir in the fresh parsley just before serving.

Sodium: Approximately 85mg | Potassium: Approximately 600mg | Phosphorus: Approximately 220mg | Protein: Approximately 34g

Snacks and Sides

When managing kidney health, every meal and snack plays a crucial role. It's essential to choose snacks and sides that not only satisfy hunger but also contribute positively to daily nutritional goals without overburdening the kidneys. For individuals following a renal diet, this means selecting foods that are low in sodium, potassium, and phosphorus while being mindful of protein intake. The right snacks and sides can provide valuable energy, essential nutrients, and the variety needed to keep meals interesting and enjoyable.

The challenge often lies in finding options that meet these criteria without compromising on taste or convenience. However, with a bit of creativity and planning, it's entirely possible to enjoy delicious and nutritious snacks and sides that support kidney health. These choices can help stabilize blood sugar levels, reduce the workload on the kidneys, and ensure that dietary restrictions do not lead to nutrient deficiencies or unwanted weight loss.

In this section, we will explore a range of snack and side dish options designed specifically for those on a renal diet. From fresh and crunchy vegetables paired with kidney-friendly dips to wholesome grains and legumes prepared with herbs and spices that pack a flavor punch without the added sodium, these recipes aim to delight the palate while nurturing the body. Whether you're looking for a quick bite between meals, a complement to your main dish, or a healthy way to satisfy a craving, these snacks and sides are tailored to fit seamlessly into a renal-friendly eating plan, ensuring you can enjoy the flavors you love while keeping your kidney health in check.

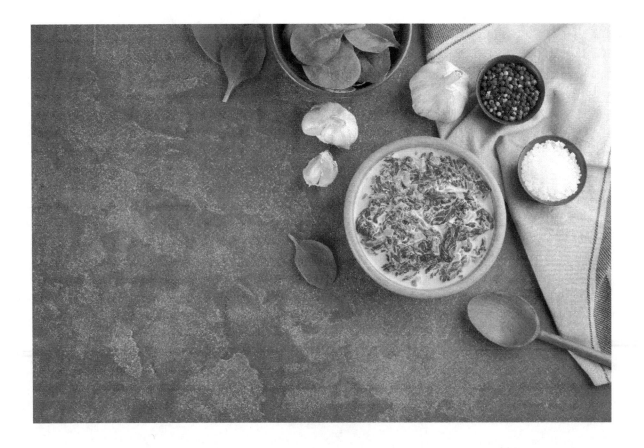

Spinach and Artichoke Dip

Preparation Time: 10 min | Cooking Time: 25 min | Serving Size: 8 servings

Ingredients

- 1 cup fresh spinach, chopped
- 1 can (14 ounces) artichoke hearts, drained and chopped
- 1 cup low-fat cream cheese
- 1/2 cup sour cream
- 1/4 cup mayonnaise
- 1 clove garlic, minced
- 1/2 cup grated Parmesan cheese
- 1/2 teaspoon ground black pepper
- Salt (optional)

Step-by-Step Cooking Instructions

Preheat Oven: Preheat your oven to 375°F (190°C).
Mix Ingredients: In a large bowl, combine the chopped spinach, artichoke hearts, low-fat cream cheese, sour cream, mayonnaise, minced garlic, grated Parmesan cheese, and black pepper. Mix until well combined. Season with optional salt to taste.
Bake: Transfer the mixture to a baking dish. Bake in the preheated oven for 20-25 minutes, or until the top is lightly golden and bubbly.
Serve: Serve warm with renal-diet-friendly sides, such as sliced bell peppers, cucumber, or homemade low-sodium pita chips.

Sodium: Approximately 180mg | Potassium: Approximately 120mg | Phosphorus: Approximately 100mg | Protein: Approximately 5g

This Spinach and Artichoke Dip recipe is a creamy and delicious option that fits perfectly into a renal-friendly diet. By incorporating low-fat cream cheese and sour cream, it reduces the overall fat content while maintaining a rich, satisfying texture. The use of fresh spinach and artichokes not only adds flavor and nutrients but also keeps the potassium and phosphorus levels in check. Parmesan cheese lends a salty bite, which can be adjusted according to dietary sodium restrictions. Whether enjoyed as an appetizer or a snack, this dip offers a way to indulge in a classic favorite without straying from kidney health guidelines.

Cheesy Cauliflower Bake

Preparation Time: 15 min | Cooking Time: 25 min | Serving Size: 6 servings

Ingredients

- 1 large head cauliflower, cut into florets
- 2 tablespoons olive oil
- Salt (optional) and pepper to taste
- 1 cup low-fat milk
- 2 tablespoons all-purpose flour
- 1 cup grated low-sodium cheddar cheese
- 1/2 teaspoon garlic powder
- 1/2 teaspoon paprika
- 1/4 cup grated Parmesan cheese
- 2 tablespoons breadcrumbs (optional)

Step-by-Step Cooking Instructions

Preheat Oven: Preheat your oven to 375°F (190°C).

Prepare Cauliflower: Toss cauliflower florets with olive oil and season with optional salt and pepper. Spread on a baking sheet and roast for about 15 minutes, or until slightly tender.

Make Cheese Sauce: In a saucepan, whisk together milk and flour over medium heat until smooth. Add cheddar cheese, garlic powder, and paprika, stirring until the cheese is melted and the sauce is thickened.

Combine: Place the roasted cauliflower in a baking dish. Pour the cheese sauce evenly over the cauliflower. Sprinkle with grated Parmesan cheese and optional breadcrumbs.

Bake: Bake for 10-15 minutes, or until the top is golden and bubbly.

Serve: Serve warm as a side dish.

Sodium: Approximately 180mg | Potassium: Approximately 320mg | Phosphorus: Approximately 190mg | Protein: Approximately 9g

Radish and Cucumber Salad

Preparation Time: 10 min | Cooking Time: 0 min | Serving Size: 4 servings

Ingredients

- 1 cup radishes, thinly sliced
- 2 cups cucumber, thinly sliced
- 1/4 cup red onion, thinly sliced
- 2 tablespoons olive oil
- 1 tablespoon apple cider vinegar
- Salt (optional) and pepper to taste
- 1 tablespoon fresh dill, chopped

Step-by-Step Cooking Instructions

Combine Vegetables: In a large bowl, mix together the radishes, cucumber, and red onion.

Dress Salad: Add the olive oil and apple cider vinegar to the vegetables. Season with optional salt and pepper, and toss to coat evenly.

Garnish: Sprinkle with fresh dill and toss again before serving.

Serve: Enjoy this refreshing salad as a light side dish.

Nutritional Information per Serving

Sodium: Approximately 30mg | Potassium: Approximately 200mg | Phosphorus: Approximately 35mg | Protein: Approximately 1g

Broccoli and Carrot Slaw

Preparation Time: 15 min | Cooking Time: 0 min | Serving Size: 4 servings

Ingredients

- 2 cups broccoli florets, finely chopped
- 1 cup carrots, shredded
- 1/4 cup red onion, finely chopped
- 2 tablespoons raisins (optional)
- 1/4 cup low-fat mayonnaise
- 2 tablespoons apple cider vinegar
- 1 tablespoon honey
- Salt (optional) and pepper to taste

Step-by-Step Cooking Instructions

Combine Vegetables: In a large bowl, mix the broccoli, carrots, red onion, and raisins (if using) until well combined.

Prepare Dressing: In a small bowl, whisk together the low-fat mayonnaise, apple cider vinegar, and honey. Season with optional salt and pepper to taste.

Dress Slaw: Pour the dressing over the vegetable mixture and toss until everything is evenly coated.

Chill: For the best flavor, refrigerate the slaw for at least 1 hour before serving.

Serve: Enjoy this colorful and crunchy slaw as a refreshing side dish.

Sodium: Approximately 70mg | Potassium: Approximately 250mg | Phosphorus: Approximately 45mg | Protein: Approximately 2g

This Broccoli and Carrot Slaw offers a vibrant and nutritious addition to any meal, especially for those adhering to a renal diet. The combination of fresh vegetables provides a rich source of vitamins and antioxidants, while the low-fat mayonnaise keeps the dish's overall fat content in check. Opting for apple cider vinegar and a touch of honey in the dressing adds a delightful sweetness and tang without overwhelming the kidneys with high levels of sodium, potassium, or phosphorus. Whether served as a standalone side or complementing a main dish, this slaw is a testament to the fact that kidney-friendly foods can be both healthful and flavorful.

Sweet Potato Hash

Preparation Time: 10 min | Cooking Time: 20 min | Serving Size: 4 servings

Ingredients

- 2 medium sweet potatoes, peeled and diced
- 1 red bell pepper, diced
- 1 small onion, diced
- 2 tablespoons olive oil
- 1/2 teaspoon smoked paprika
- Salt (optional) and pepper to taste
- 2 tablespoons fresh parsley, chopped (for garnish)

Step-by-Step Cooking Instructions

Prepare Ingredients: In a large bowl, combine diced sweet potatoes, red bell pepper, and onion. Drizzle with olive oil and season with smoked paprika, and optional salt and pepper. Toss to coat evenly.

Cook Hash: Heat a large skillet over medium-high heat. Add the vegetable mixture to the skillet, spreading it out into an even layer. Cook for about 10 minutes, stirring occasionally, until the vegetables start to soften.

Brown Hash: Reduce the heat to medium and continue cooking, stirring occasionally, for another 10 minutes, or until the sweet potatoes are tender and lightly browned.

Garnish and Serve: Remove from heat, garnish with fresh parsley, and serve immediately.

Sodium: Approximately 75mg | Potassium: Approximately 450mg | Phosphorus: Approximately 100mg | Protein: Approximately 2g

Stuffed Bell Peppers with Rice and Herbs

Preparation Time: 20 min | Cooking Time: 30 min | Serving Size: 4 servings

Ingredients

- 4 large bell peppers, tops removed and seeds cleaned out
- 1 cup cooked rice
- 1 tablespoon olive oil
- 1 small onion, finely chopped
- 2 cloves garlic, minced
- 1 tomato, diced
- 1/4 cup fresh parsley, chopped
- 1/4 cup fresh basil, chopped
- Salt (optional) and pepper to taste
- 1/4 cup low-sodium vegetable broth

Step-by-Step Cooking Instructions

Preheat Oven: Preheat your oven to 350°F (175°C).
Prepare Filling: In a skillet over medium heat, heat olive oil. Add onion and garlic, cooking until soft. Add the cooked rice, diced tomato, parsley, and basil. Season with optional salt and pepper. Cook for another 5 minutes, stirring occasionally.
Stuff Peppers: Spoon the rice and herb mixture into each bell pepper. Place the stuffed peppers upright in a baking dish.
Bake: Pour the vegetable broth into the bottom of the dish. Cover with foil and bake for about 30 minutes, or until the peppers are tender.
Serve: Serve the stuffed bell peppers warm.

Sodium: Approximately 80mg | Potassium: Approximately 300mg | Phosphorus: Approximately 100mg | Protein: Approximately 4g

Pineapple Cucumber Salad

Preparation Time: 10 min | Cooking Time: 0 min | Serving Size: 4 servings

Ingredients

- 2 cups fresh pineapple, diced
- 1 large cucumber, diced
- 1/4 cup red onion, finely sliced
- 1 tablespoon lime juice
- 1 tablespoon olive oil
- 1/2 teaspoon chili powder (optional)
- Salt (optional) and pepper to taste
- 2 tablespoons fresh cilantro, chopped

Step-by-Step Cooking Instructions

Combine Salad Ingredients: In a large bowl, mix together the diced pineapple, cucumber, and sliced red onion.

Dress the Salad: Add lime juice and olive oil to the bowl. Sprinkle with chili powder (if using), and season with optional salt and pepper. Toss everything together until well combined.

Garnish: Sprinkle chopped cilantro over the salad and give it one final toss.

Serve: Enjoy this refreshing salad as a light side dish or a palate cleanser between meals.

Nutritional Information per Serving

Sodium: Approximately 10mg | Potassium: Approximately 180mg | Phosphorus: Approximately 20mg | Protein: Approximately 1g

Edamame Salad

Preparation Time: 15 min | Cooking Time: 0 min | Serving Size: 4 servings

Ingredients

- 2 cups cooked edamame, shelled
- 1 red bell pepper, diced
- 1 carrot, julienned or shredded
- 1/4 cup red onion, finely chopped
- 2 tablespoons fresh cilantro, chopped
- 2 tablespoons rice vinegar
- 1 tablespoon sesame oil
- 1 teaspoon honey
- Salt (optional) and pepper to taste
- 1 teaspoon sesame seeds (for garnish)

Step-by-Step Cooking Instructions

Mix Salad Ingredients: In a large bowl, combine the edamame, red bell pepper, carrot, red onion, and cilantro.

Prepare Dressing: In a small bowl, whisk together the rice vinegar, sesame oil, and honey. Season with optional salt and pepper.

Combine: Pour the dressing over the salad and toss to coat evenly.

Garnish: Sprinkle sesame seeds over the top of the salad.

Chill & Serve: For the best flavor, let the salad chill in the refrigerator for at least 1 hour before serving. Enjoy it cold.

Sodium: Approximately 55mg | Potassium: Approximately 500mg | Phosphorus: Approximately 150mg | Protein: Approximately 11g

Baked Garlic Parmesan Zucchini Chips

Preparation Time: 10 min | Cooking Time: 20 min | Serving Size: 4 servings

Ingredients

- 2 medium zucchinis, thinly sliced
- 1 tablespoon olive oil
- 1/2 cup grated Parmesan cheese
- 1 teaspoon garlic powder
- Salt (optional) and pepper to taste
- 1 teaspoon dried oregano

Step-by-Step Cooking Instructions

Preheat Oven: Preheat your oven to 425°F (220°C). Line a baking sheet with parchment paper.

Prepare Zucchini: In a large bowl, toss the zucchini slices with olive oil, garlic powder, optional salt, and pepper until evenly coated.

Coat Zucchini: Place the zucchini slices in a single layer on the prepared baking sheet. Sprinkle grated Parmesan cheese and dried oregano over the zucchini slices.

Bake: Bake in the preheated oven for about 20 minutes, or until the zucchini is crispy and the cheese is golden brown.

Serve: Enjoy the zucchini chips hot as a delicious and healthy snack or side dish.

Sodium: Approximately 180mg | Potassium: Approximately 250mg | Phosphorus: Approximately 100mg | Protein: Approximately 7g

These Baked Garlic Parmesan Zucchini Chips are a kidney-friendly alternative to traditional snacks, providing a delightful crunch with far less sodium and unhealthy fats. The combination of zucchini, rich in vitamins and minerals, with the savory flavor of Parmesan cheese and garlic, creates a snack that's not only tasty but also nutritious. Opting for baking instead of frying transforms this dish into a healthier choice that supports renal health. With careful attention to the nutritional content, especially the sodium, potassium, and phosphorus levels, these chips offer a guilt-free way to satisfy those snack cravings while adhering to a renal diet.

Parmesan Roasted Asparagus

Preparation Time: 5 min | Cooking Time: 15 min | Serving Size: 4 servings

Ingredients

- 1 pound asparagus, ends trimmed
- 2 tablespoons olive oil
- 1/4 cup grated Parmesan cheese
- Salt (optional) and pepper to taste
- 1 teaspoon garlic powder

Step-by-Step Cooking Instructions

Preheat Oven: Preheat your oven to 400°F (200°C). Line a baking sheet with parchment paper.

Prepare Asparagus: Place the asparagus on the prepared baking sheet. Drizzle with olive oil and toss to coat evenly. Season with garlic powder, and optional salt and pepper.

Add Parmesan: Sprinkle grated Parmesan cheese over the asparagus.

Roast: Bake in the preheated oven for about 15 minutes, or until the asparagus is tender and the cheese is lightly golden.

Serve: Enjoy the Parmesan roasted asparagus hot as a flavorful and nutritious side dish.

Sodium: Approximately 115mg | Potassium: Approximately 230mg | Phosphorus: Approximately 75mg | Protein: Approximately 5g

Parmesan Roasted Asparagus is a simple, elegant side dish that brings out the natural flavors of asparagus with the delicious addition of Parmesan cheese. This recipe is designed with a renal diet in mind, ensuring low sodium, potassium, and phosphorus content while providing a good source of protein. The olive oil and garlic powder enhance the asparagus's taste without needing excessive salt, making it a healthy choice for those managing kidney health. The golden, crispy Parmesan topping adds a delightful texture and savory note to the tender asparagus, making it a perfect accompaniment to a variety of main dishes.

Roasted Pumpkin Seeds

Preparation Time: 10 min | Cooking Time: 45 min | Serving Size: 4 servings

Ingredients

- 1 cup raw pumpkin seeds, cleaned and dried
- 1 tablespoon olive oil
- Salt (optional) to taste
- 1/2 teaspoon paprika (optional)
- 1/2 teaspoon garlic powder (optional)

Step-by-Step Cooking Instructions

Preheat Oven: Preheat your oven to 300°F (150°C). Line a baking sheet with parchment paper.
Prepare Seeds: In a bowl, toss the pumpkin seeds with olive oil, optional salt, paprika, and garlic powder until evenly coated.
Roast Seeds: Spread the seeds in a single layer on the prepared baking sheet. Roast in the preheated oven for about 45 minutes, stirring occasionally, until golden and crunchy.
Cool & Serve: Let the seeds cool before serving. Enjoy as a crunchy, nutritious snack.

Sodium: Approximately 5mg | Potassium: Approximately 129mg | Phosphorus: Approximately 333mg | Protein: Approximately 7g

Roasted Pumpkin Seeds are a savory, crunchy snack that fits well into a renal diet when sodium intake is carefully managed. These seeds are a great source of protein and phosphorus, with a moderate amount of potassium. The optional seasonings of paprika and garlic powder add flavor without the need for excess salt, making them a healthier option for those monitoring their sodium consumption. This snack is not only delicious but also packed with nutrients that support kidney health, offering a satisfying crunch that's both nutritious and enjoyable.

Zucchini Fritters

Preparation Time: 15 min | Cooking Time: 10 min | Serving Size: 4 servings

Ingredients

- 2 medium zucchinis, grated
- 1/4 cup all-purpose flour
- 1/4 cup grated low-sodium Parmesan cheese
- 1 egg, beaten
- 2 tablespoons chives, finely chopped
- Salt (optional) and pepper to taste
- 2 tablespoons olive oil for frying

Step-by-Step Cooking Instructions

Drain Zucchini: Place the grated zucchini in a colander, sprinkle with optional salt, and let sit for 10 minutes. Squeeze out the excess water.
Mix Ingredients: In a large bowl, combine the drained zucchini, all-purpose flour, grated Parmesan, beaten egg, and chives. Season with pepper and mix well.
Form Fritters: Heat olive oil in a large skillet over medium heat. Scoop tablespoons of the zucchini mixture into the skillet, flattening them into small patties.
Cook Fritters: Fry for about 5 minutes on each side, or until golden brown and crispy.
Serve: Serve the zucchini fritters hot, with a side of low-sodium sour cream or yogurt if desired.

Sodium: Approximately 80mg | Potassium: Approximately 250mg | Phosphorus: Approximately 100mg | Protein: Approximately 6g

Carrot and Celery Sticks with Ranch Dip (Renal-Friendly Version)

Preparation Time: 10 min | Cooking Time: 0 min | Serving Size: 4 servings

Ingredients

For the Dip:

- 1/2 cup low-fat sour cream
- 1/4 cup mayonnaise (low-sodium)
- 1 tablespoon fresh dill, chopped
- 1 tablespoon fresh parsley, chopped
- 1 clove garlic, minced
- 1/2 teaspoon onion powder
- Salt (optional) and pepper to taste

For the Sticks:

- 2 large carrots, peeled and cut into sticks
- 2 large celery stalks, cut into sticks

Step-by-Step Cooking Instructions

Prepare Ranch Dip: In a bowl, mix together the low-fat sour cream, low-sodium mayonnaise, chopped dill, parsley, minced garlic, and onion powder. Season with optional salt and pepper to taste. Refrigerate until ready to serve.
Prepare Vegetable Sticks: Cut the carrots and celery into stick shapes suitable for dipping.
Serve: Serve the carrot and celery sticks with the ranch dip on the side.

Sodium: Approximately 70mg | Potassium: Approximately 200mg | Phosphorus: Approximately 60mg | Protein: Approximately 2g

Fruit Salad with Mint

Preparation Time: 15 min | Cooking Time: 0 min | Serving Size: 4 servings

Ingredients

- 1 cup strawberries, hulled and halved
- 1 cup blueberries
- 1 cup grapes, halved
- 2 kiwis, peeled and sliced
- 1/2 cup pineapple, diced
- 2 tablespoons fresh mint, chopped
- Juice of 1 lemon

Step-by-Step Cooking Instructions

Combine Fruits: In a large bowl, gently mix together the strawberries, blueberries, grapes, kiwis, and pineapple.
Add Flavor: Sprinkle the chopped mint over the fruit. Drizzle with lemon juice and toss lightly to combine.
Chill & Serve: Refrigerate the salad for at least 1 hour before serving to allow flavors to meld. Serve chilled.

Sodium: Approximately 5mg | Potassium: Approximately 250mg | Phosphorus: Approximately 50mg | Protein: Approximately 2g

This Fruit Salad with Mint is a refreshing, kidney-friendly dessert or snack that combines the natural sweetness of various fruits with the cool, refreshing taste of mint and the bright acidity of lemon juice. This mix not only provides a delicious variety of flavors and textures but also a good balance of nutrients. The selection of fruits is designed to be mindful of potassium and phosphorus levels, making this salad suitable for those on a renal diet. The addition of mint and lemon enhances the natural flavors of the fruits without the need for added sugars or artificial ingredients, creating a healthful and hydrating option for any time of the day.

Baked Kale Chips

Preparation Time: 10 min | Cooking Time: 15 min | Serving Size: 4 servings

Ingredients

- 1 bunch kale, washed and dried
- 1 tablespoon olive oil
- Salt (optional) to taste
- 1 teaspoon garlic powder

Step-by-Step Cooking Instructions

Preheat Oven: Preheat your oven to 350°F (175°C). Line a baking sheet with parchment paper.

Prepare Kale: Remove the kale leaves from the stems and tear into bite-sized pieces. Place the kale pieces in a large bowl.

Season Kale: Drizzle olive oil over the kale. Add garlic powder and optional salt. Toss until the kale pieces are evenly coated.

Bake: Spread the kale pieces in a single layer on the prepared baking sheet. Bake in the preheated oven for about 15 minutes, or until the edges are slightly browned and crisp, turning halfway through.

Serve: Let the kale chips cool slightly before serving. Enjoy as a crunchy, nutritious snack.

Sodium: Approximately 30mg | Potassium: Approximately 300mg | Phosphorus: Approximately 50mg | Protein: Approximately 2g

Italian-inspired Tomato and Basil Bruschetta

Preparation Time: 15 min | Cooking Time: 5 min | Serving Size: 4 servings

Ingredients

- 4 slices of whole grain bread, toasted
- 2 large tomatoes, diced
- 1/4 cup fresh basil leaves, chopped
- 1 tablespoon olive oil
- 1 clove garlic, minced
- Salt (optional) and pepper to taste
- 1 tablespoon balsamic vinegar (optional)

Step-by-Step Cooking Instructions

Toast Bread: Toast the whole grain bread slices until they are crisp and golden.
Prepare Topping: In a bowl, combine the diced tomatoes, chopped basil, olive oil, and minced garlic. Season with optional salt and pepper. If desired, add balsamic vinegar for a touch of sweetness and acidity.
Assemble Bruschetta: Spoon the tomato and basil mixture generously onto each slice of toasted bread.
Serve: Serve immediately while the bread is still crisp for the best texture contrast.

Sodium: Approximately 70mg | Potassium: Approximately 200mg | Phosphorus: Approximately 60mg | Protein: Approximately 4g

This Italian-inspired Tomato and Basil Bruschetta is a light and flavorful appetizer that captures the essence of Italian cuisine while being mindful of a renal diet. Fresh tomatoes and basil provide a burst of freshness and are a good source of vitamins without adding excessive potassium. The whole grain bread adds a satisfying crunch and fiber, making this dish not only delicious but also nutritious. By using olive oil and optional balsamic vinegar, you enhance the flavors without the need for high sodium content, making it a suitable choice for those managing kidney health. Enjoy this classic Italian appetizer with the assurance that it is both kidney-friendly and delectably wholesome.

Garlic Roasted Cauliflower

Preparation Time: 10 min | Cooking Time: 25 min | Serving Size: 4 servings

Ingredients

- 1 large head of cauliflower, cut into florets
- 3 tablespoons olive oil
- 3 cloves garlic, minced
- Salt (optional) and pepper to taste
- 1 tablespoon fresh parsley, chopped (for garnish)

Step-by-Step Cooking Instructions

Preheat Oven: Preheat your oven to 425°F (220°C). Line a baking sheet with parchment paper.
Season Cauliflower: In a large bowl, toss cauliflower florets with olive oil, minced garlic, and optional salt and pepper until well coated.
Roast: Spread the cauliflower in a single layer on the prepared baking sheet. Roast for 25 minutes, or until tender and golden brown, stirring halfway through.
Garnish and Serve: Sprinkle roasted cauliflower with fresh parsley before serving. Enjoy as a flavorful side dish.

Sodium: Approximately 30mg | Potassium: Approximately 320mg | Phosphorus: Approximately 45mg | Protein: Approximately 3g

Garlic Roasted Cauliflower is a simple yet delicious dish that transforms a humble vegetable into a flavorful, golden delight. By roasting cauliflower with garlic and olive oil, this recipe enhances the vegetable's natural sweetness and brings out a rich, nutty flavor. This dish is carefully seasoned to ensure it remains low in sodium, making it a suitable choice for those on a renal diet. The addition of fresh parsley not only adds a burst of color but also a fresh flavor that complements the roasted garlic. With its low phosphorus and moderate potassium content, this recipe offers a kidney-friendly way to enjoy a nutritious vegetable, making it an excellent addition to any meal.

Mexican-inspired Black Bean and Corn Salad

Preparation Time: 15 min | Cooking Time: 0 min | Serving Size: 4 servings

Ingredients

- 1 cup low-sodium canned black beans, rinsed and drained
- 1 cup cooked corn kernels, cooled
- 1 red bell pepper, diced
- 1/4 cup red onion, finely chopped
- 2 tablespoons fresh cilantro, chopped
- Juice of 1 lime
- 1 tablespoon olive oil
- Salt (optional) and pepper to taste
- 1 avocado, diced (optional)

Step-by-Step Cooking Instructions

Combine Ingredients: In a large bowl, mix together the black beans, corn, red bell pepper, red onion, and cilantro.

Dress the Salad: Add lime juice and olive oil to the salad. Season with optional salt and pepper. Toss well to combine.

Add Avocado: If using, gently fold in the diced avocado right before serving.

Serve: Enjoy this vibrant salad as a refreshing side dish or a light main course.

Sodium: Approximately 100mg | Potassium: Approximately 400mg | Phosphorus: Approximately 150mg | Protein: Approximately 6g

Hummus with Cucumber Sticks

Preparation Time: 10 min | Cooking Time: 0 min | Serving Size: 4 servings

Ingredients

For the Hummus:

- 1 can (15 ounces) low-sodium chickpeas, rinsed and drained
- 2 tablespoons tahini (sesame paste)
- 2 cloves garlic, minced
- Juice of 1 lemon
- 2 tablespoons olive oil
- Salt (optional) and pepper to taste

For the Cucumber Sticks:

- 2 large cucumbers, peeled and cut into sticks

Step-by-Step Cooking Instructions

Prepare Hummus: In a food processor, blend the chickpeas, tahini, minced garlic, lemon juice, and olive oil until smooth. Season with optional salt and pepper to taste.
Prepare Cucumber Sticks: Peel cucumbers and cut them into stick shapes suitable for dipping.
Serve: Place the hummus in a serving bowl and arrange the cucumber sticks around it for dipping.

Sodium: Approximately 100mg | Potassium: Approximately 200mg | Phosphorus: Approximately 120mg | Protein: Approximately 6g

Kale Chips

Preparation Time: 10 min | Cooking Time: 20 min | Serving Size: 4 servings

Ingredients

- 1 bunch kale, tough stems removed, leaves torn into bite-sized pieces
- 1 tablespoon olive oil
- Salt (optional) to taste

Step-by-Step Cooking Instructions

Preheat Oven: Preheat your oven to 300°F (150°C). Line a baking sheet with parchment paper.

Prepare Kale: Wash and dry the kale leaves thoroughly. In a large bowl, toss the kale with olive oil and optional salt until evenly coated.

Arrange Kale: Spread the kale in a single layer on the prepared baking sheet, making sure the leaves don't overlap.

Bake: Bake in the preheated oven for about 20 minutes, or until the edges are crisp but not burnt, turning the leaves halfway through the cooking time.

Serve: Let the kale chips cool on the baking sheet before serving. Enjoy as a crunchy, healthy snack.

Sodium: Approximately 25mg | Potassium: Approximately 491mg | Phosphorus: Approximately 92mg | Protein: Approximately 3g

Kale Chips are a nutritious and delicious alternative to traditional snack chips, offering a renal-friendly option for those managing their kidney health. This recipe uses minimal ingredients to highlight the natural flavors and nutritional benefits of kale, including vitamins, minerals, and fiber. By opting for olive oil and controlling the addition of salt, these kale chips provide a lower sodium snack compared to store-bought alternatives. The careful preparation and baking process ensure a crispy texture that satisfies the craving for something crunchy. Enjoy these kale chips as a guilt-free snack that supports your dietary needs without compromising on taste.

Apple Cinnamon Muffins

Preparation Time: 15 min | Cooking Time: 20 min | Serving Size: 12 muffins

Ingredients

- 1 1/2 cups all-purpose flour
- 1/2 cup sugar
- 2 teaspoons baking powder (low-sodium)
- 1/2 teaspoon baking soda
- 2 teaspoons cinnamon
- 1/4 teaspoon salt (optional)
- 3/4 cup unsweetened applesauce
- 1/4 cup vegetable oil
- 1 egg
- 1 cup finely chopped apples

Step-by-Step Cooking Instructions

Preheat Oven: Preheat your oven to 350°F (175°C). Line a muffin tin with paper liners or lightly grease it.

Mix Dry Ingredients: In a large bowl, combine the flour, sugar, baking powder, baking soda, cinnamon, and optional salt.

Add Wet Ingredients: Stir in the applesauce, vegetable oil, and egg until just combined. Fold in the chopped apples.

Fill Muffin Tin: Divide the batter evenly among the prepared muffin cups.

Bake: Bake in the preheated oven for 20 minutes, or until a toothpick inserted into the center of a muffin comes out clean.

Cool and Serve: Let the muffins cool in the pan for 5 minutes, then transfer to a wire rack to cool completely.

Sodium: Approximately 95mg | Potassium: Approximately 60mg | Phosphorus: Approximately 50mg | Protein: Approximately 2g

Desserts and Treats

When following a renal diet, addressing the craving for sweets might seem challenging at first. The key to indulging in desserts and treats lies in moderation and smart substitutions, ensuring that you can enjoy these pleasures without compromising your health. Renal diets often require restrictions on certain nutrients such as potassium, phosphorus, sodium, and sometimes fluid intake. However, with a little creativity and careful planning, you can satisfy your sweet tooth while adhering to these dietary guidelines.

Understanding which ingredients to limit or avoid is crucial in preparing kidney-friendly desserts. For example, certain dairy products high in phosphorus or fruits rich in potassium might need to be consumed in moderation or substituted with lower-potassium alternatives. Similarly, reducing the sodium and sugar content in desserts can help manage blood pressure and blood sugar levels, contributing to overall kidney health and well-being.

The art of renal-friendly dessert making involves using ingredients like low-phosphorus dairy substitutes, fruits low in potassium, and incorporating herbs and spices for flavor without the added salt or sugar. Flour alternatives, such as almond or coconut flour, can be used for baking to lower the phosphorus content, while herbs like mint or cinnamon can add a burst of flavor without compromising dietary restrictions.

In this section, we will explore a variety of dessert and treat recipes that are both delicious and kidney-friendly. From creamy puddings and light, fruit-based desserts to savory baked goods made with kidney-safe ingredients, these recipes are designed to bring joy and satisfaction without the guilt. So, let's dive into the world of renal diet-friendly desserts, where moderation and smart substitutions open the door to a wide array of sweet possibilities.

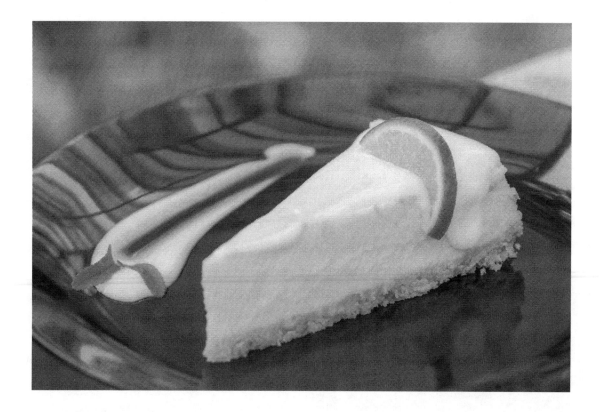

Key Lime Pie

Preparation Time: 20 min | Cooking Time: 10 min + chilling time | Serving Size: 8 servings

Ingredients

- **Crust:**
    - 1 1/2 cups graham cracker crumbs (low-sodium)
    - 1/3 cup unsalted butter, melted
    - 3 tablespoons sugar
- **Filling:**
    - 1 can (14 ounces) low-fat sweetened condensed milk
    - 1/2 cup key lime juice
    - 1 teaspoon lime zest
    - 2 egg yolks
- **Topping:**
    - 1 cup heavy whipping cream
    - 1 tablespoon powdered sugar

Step-by-Step Cooking Instructions

Prepare Crust: Mix graham cracker crumbs, melted butter, and sugar in a bowl. Press mixture firmly into the bottom and up the sides of a 9-inch pie plate. Bake at 350°F (175°C) for 10 minutes. Cool completely.

Make Filling: Whisk together sweetened condensed milk, key lime juice, lime zest, and egg yolks until smooth. Pour into cooled crust.

Chill: Refrigerate pie for at least 4 hours, or until set.

Prepare Topping: Before serving, whip heavy cream and powdered sugar until stiff peaks form. Spread over the pie.

Serve: Garnish with additional lime zest if desired. Serve chilled.

Sodium: Approximately 120mg | Potassium: Approximately 150mg | Phosphorus: Approximately 100mg | Protein: Approximately 5g

Apple Crisp

Preparation Time: 15 min | Cooking Time: 45 min | Serving Size: 6 servings

Ingredients

- **Filling:**
    - 4 cups sliced apples (peeled)
    - 1/2 teaspoon cinnamon
    - 1/4 cup sugar
- **Topping:**
    - 3/4 cup rolled oats
    - 1/3 cup all-purpose flour
    - 1/2 cup brown sugar, packed
    - 1/2 teaspoon cinnamon
    - 1/4 cup unsalted butter, softened

Step-by-Step Cooking Instructions

Preheat Oven: Preheat your oven to 350°F (175°C). Grease an 8-inch square baking dish.

Prepare Filling: In a large bowl, toss the sliced apples with cinnamon and sugar. Spread the apple mixture evenly in the prepared baking dish.

Make Topping: In another bowl, mix together the rolled oats, flour, brown sugar, and cinnamon. Cut in the butter until the mixture resembles coarse crumbs. Sprinkle this topping over the apples.

Bake: Place the baking dish in the preheated oven and bake for about 45 minutes, or until the topping is golden brown and the apples are tender.

Serve: Allow the apple crisp to cool slightly before serving. Enjoy warm.

Sodium: Approximately 5mg | Potassium: Approximately 150mg | Phosphorus: Approximately 50mg | Protein: Approximately 2g

Pumpkin Pie with Whipped Cream

Preparation Time: 20 min | Cooking Time: 55 min | Serving Size: 8 servings

Ingredients

- **Pie:**
    - 1 (9-inch) unbaked pie crust (low-sodium)
    - 2 cups pumpkin puree
    - 3/4 cup sugar
    - 1/2 teaspoon salt (optional)
    - 1 teaspoon ground cinnamon
    - 1/2 teaspoon ground ginger
    - 1/4 teaspoon ground cloves
    - 2 large eggs
    - 1 cup evaporated milk
- **Whipped Cream:**
    - 1 cup heavy whipping cream
    - 1 tablespoon powdered sugar

Step-by-Step Cooking Instructions

Preheat Oven: Preheat your oven to 425°F (220°C).
Mix Filling: In a large bowl, combine pumpkin puree, sugar, optional salt, cinnamon, ginger, and cloves. Add eggs and mix well. Gradually stir in evaporated milk.
Prepare Pie: Pour the filling into the unbaked pie crust.
Bake: Bake for 15 minutes. Reduce the oven temperature to 350°F (175°C) and continue baking for 40 minutes, or until a knife inserted near the center comes out clean.
Cool: Allow the pie to cool on a wire rack.
Make Whipped Cream: Beat heavy whipping cream and powdered sugar until stiff peaks form.
Serve: Serve each slice of pumpkin pie with a dollop of whipped cream.

Sodium: Approximately 150mg | Potassium: Approximately 200mg | Phosphorus: Approximately 100mg | Protein: Approximately 5g

Strawberry Shortcake

Preparation Time: 20 min | Cooking Time: 15 min | Serving Size: 8 servings

Ingredients

- **Shortcakes:**
    - 2 cups all-purpose flour
    - 3 tablespoons sugar
    - 1 tablespoon baking powder (low-sodium)
    - 1/2 teaspoon salt (optional)
    - 1/3 cup cold unsalted butter, cubed
    - 3/4 cup low-fat milk
- **Strawberries:**
    - 4 cups strawberries, sliced
    - 1/4 cup sugar
- **Whipped Cream:**
    - 1 cup heavy whipping cream
    - 1 tablespoon powdered sugar

Step-by-Step Cooking Instructions

Preheat Oven: Preheat your oven to 425°F (220°C). Line a baking sheet with parchment paper.
Make Shortcake Dough: In a large bowl, combine flour, sugar, baking powder, and optional salt. Cut in butter until mixture resembles coarse crumbs. Gradually stir in milk until dough forms.
Shape Shortcakes: Drop dough by spoonfuls onto the prepared baking sheet, forming 8 shortcakes. Bake for 15 minutes or until golden brown. Remove from oven and let cool.
Prepare Strawberries: In a bowl, toss sliced strawberries with sugar. Set aside to macerate for at least 30 minutes.
Make Whipped Cream: Beat heavy cream and powdered sugar until stiff peaks form.
Assemble Strawberry Shortcakes: Split each shortcake in half horizontally. Spoon some of the strawberries and their juice onto the bottom half. Add a dollop of whipped cream, then cap with the top half of the shortcake. Finish with a small dollop of whipped cream and a few strawberry slices.

Sodium: Approximately 75mg | Potassium: Approximately 200mg | Phosphorus: Approximately 100mg | Protein: Approximately 4g

This Strawberry Shortcake recipe is tailored for those following a renal diet, focusing on lower sodium and moderate potassium and phosphorus levels. The use of low-sodium baking powder, optional salt, and unsalted butter helps minimize the sodium content. Strawberries provide a natural sweetness and are a good source of vitamins without significantly increasing the potassium content when consumed in moderation. The homemade whipped cream adds a luxurious finish without excessive phosphorus, making this a delightful dessert that balances indulgence with dietary management. Enjoy this classic treat that brings the essence of spring and summer into a kidney-friendly dessert.

Chocolate Chip Cookies (Kidney-Friendly)

Preparation Time: 15 min | Cooking Time: 10 min | Serving Size: 24 cookies

Ingredients

- 2 cups all-purpose flour
- 1/2 teaspoon baking soda (low-sodium)
- 1/4 teaspoon salt (optional)
- 3/4 cup unsalted butter, melted
- 1 cup brown sugar
- 1/2 cup white sugar
- 1 tablespoon vanilla extract
- 1 egg
- 1 egg yolk
- 2 cups chocolate chips (low-sodium)

Step-by-Step Cooking Instructions

Preheat Oven: Preheat your oven to 325°F (165°C). Line cookie sheets with parchment paper.

Combine Dry Ingredients: In a bowl, sift together the flour, baking soda, and optional salt.

Mix Wet Ingredients: In another bowl, cream together the melted butter, brown sugar, and white sugar until well blended. Beat in the vanilla, egg, and egg yolk until light and creamy. Mix in the sifted ingredients until just blended. Stir in the chocolate chips by hand using a wooden spoon.

Shape Cookies: Drop cookie dough 1/4 cup at a time onto the prepared cookie sheets. Cookies should be about 3 inches apart.

Bake: Bake for 10-12 minutes in the preheated oven, or until the edges are lightly toasted. Cool on baking sheets for a few minutes before transferring to wire racks to cool completely.

Sodium: Approximately 20mg | Potassium: Approximately 50mg | Phosphorus: Approximately 25mg | Protein: Approximately 2g

Banana Ice Cream

Preparation Time: 10 min | Cooking Time: 0 min (Freezing time: 2 hours) | Serving Size: 4 servings

Ingredients

- 4 ripe bananas, sliced and frozen

Optional Flavor Add-ins

- 1 teaspoon vanilla extract
- 2 tablespoons peanut butter (unsalted)
- 2 tablespoons cocoa powder (for chocolate flavor)

Step-by-Step Cooking Instructions

Prepare Bananas: Peel and slice bananas. Freeze the slices for at least 2 hours or until solid.

Blend Bananas: Place the frozen banana slices into a food processor. Blend until smooth and creamy. This may take a few minutes, and you might need to scrape down the sides of the bowl occasionally.

Flavor (Optional): Once the bananas have a creamy consistency, add any optional flavor add-ins like vanilla extract, peanut butter, or cocoa powder. Blend until well combined.

Serve or Freeze: Serve immediately for a soft-serve texture, or transfer to a freezer-safe container and freeze for an additional hour for a firmer ice cream consistency.

Enjoy: Serve your banana ice cream in bowls. It can be garnished with fresh fruit or a sprinkle of cinnamon if desired.

Sodium: Approximately 1mg | Potassium: Approximately 422mg | Phosphorus: Approximately 34mg | Protein: Approximately 1.3g

Raspberry Gelatin

Preparation Time: 10 min | Cooking Time: 0 min + 4 hours chilling | Serving Size: 6 servings

Ingredients

- 2 cups boiling water
- 1 packet unsweetened raspberry gelatin mix (low-sodium, if available)
- 2 cups cold water
- 1 cup fresh raspberries

Step-by-Step Cooking Instructions

Dissolve Gelatin: In a large bowl, stir the boiling water and gelatin mix until completely dissolved.

Add Cold Water: Stir in the cold water.

Add Raspberries: Gently fold in the fresh raspberries.

Chill: Pour the mixture into a gelatin mold or individual serving dishes. Refrigerate for at least 4 hours, or until set.

Serve: Once set, enjoy this refreshing and light dessert.

Nutritional Information per Serving

Sodium: Approximately 10mg | Potassium: Approximately 60mg | Phosphorus: Approximately 15mg | Protein: Approximately 2g

This Raspberry Gelatin recipe offers a kidney-friendly dessert option that's both delicious and easy to make. By using unsweetened gelatin mix and fresh raspberries, this dessert keeps sodium, potassium, and phosphorus levels low, making it suitable for those on a renal diet. The fresh raspberries not only provide natural sweetness and flavor but also add a nutritional boost with their antioxidants and vitamins. This light and refreshing dessert is perfect for satisfying sweet cravings without compromising dietary restrictions, making it a great choice for any time you desire something sweet and satisfying.

Baked Peaches with Honey and Cinnamon

Preparation Time: 10 minutes | Cooking Time: 25 minutes | Serving Size: 2 servings

Ingredients:

- 2 ripe peaches, halved and pitted
- 2 tablespoons honey
- 1/2 teaspoon ground cinnamon
- Optional: chopped nuts or Greek yogurt for serving

Instructions:

Preheat your oven to 375°F (190°C).
Place the peach halves, cut side up, in a baking dish.
Drizzle honey over each peach half, then sprinkle with ground cinnamon.
Bake in the preheated oven for about 25 minutes or until the peaches are tender and caramelized.
Serve warm, optionally topped with chopped nuts or a dollop of Greek yogurt.

Calories: 120 | Total Fat: 0.5g | Sodium: 0mg | Potassium: 240mg | Total Carbohydrates: 30g | Dietary Fiber: 3g | Sugars: 26g | Protein: 1g

Coconut Rice Pudding

Preparation Time: 5 minutes | Cooking Time: 35 minutes | Serving Size: 4 servings

Ingredients:

- 1 cup white rice
- 2 cups water
- 1 (13.5 oz) can coconut milk
- 1/4 cup honey or sweetener of choice
- 1 teaspoon vanilla extract
- 1/4 teaspoon ground cinnamon
- Optional toppings: fresh fruit, chopped nuts, or shredded coconut

Instructions:

In a saucepan, combine the rice and water. Bring to a boil, then reduce heat to low, cover, and simmer for 15 minutes.

Stir in the coconut milk, honey, vanilla extract, and ground cinnamon.

Continue to cook, uncovered, over low heat for an additional 20 minutes, stirring occasionally, until the rice is tender and the mixture has thickened.

Remove from heat and let the pudding cool slightly before serving.

Serve warm or chilled, topped with your choice of fresh fruit, chopped nuts, or shredded coconut.

Calories: 300 | Total Fat: 15g | Sodium: 10mg | Potassium: 180mg | Total Carbohydrates: 40g | Dietary Fiber: 1g | Sugars: 15g | Protein: 3g

Pear and Berry Crumble

Preparation Time: 15 minutes | Cooking Time: 40 minutes | Serving Size: 6 servings

Ingredients:

- 4 ripe pears, peeled, cored, and sliced
- 1 cup mixed berries (such as strawberries, blueberries, raspberries)
- 1 tablespoon lemon juice
- 1/4 cup honey or sweetener of choice
- 1/2 teaspoon ground cinnamon
- 1/2 cup old-fashioned oats
- 1/4 cup almond flour
- 1/4 cup chopped nuts (such as almonds or walnuts)
- 2 tablespoons coconut oil, melted

Instructions:

Preheat your oven to 350°F (175°C).

In a mixing bowl, combine the sliced pears, mixed berries, lemon juice, honey, and ground cinnamon. Toss to coat the fruit evenly.

Transfer the fruit mixture to a baking dish.

In another bowl, mix together the oats, almond flour, chopped nuts, and melted coconut oil until well combined.

Spread the oat mixture evenly over the fruit in the baking dish.

Bake in the preheated oven for about 40 minutes or until the fruit is bubbling and the topping is golden brown.

Allow the crumble to cool slightly before serving.

Serve warm, optionally topped with a dollop of Greek yogurt or a drizzle of honey.

Calories: 220 | Total Fat: 9g | Sodium: 0mg | Potassium: 250mg | Total Carbohydrates: 36g | Dietary Fiber: 6g | Sugars: 20g | Protein: 3g

Fruit Sorbet

Preparation Time: 10 minutes | Freezing Time: 4 hours | Serving Size: 4 servings

Ingredients:

- 2 cups frozen mixed fruit (such as berries, mango, pineapple)
- 1 ripe banana, peeled and frozen
- 2 tablespoons honey or sweetener of choice
- 1/4 cup water
- Optional: fresh mint leaves for garnish

Instructions:

In a blender or food processor, combine the frozen mixed fruit, frozen banana, honey, and water.

Blend until smooth and creamy, scraping down the sides as needed.

If the mixture is too thick, add a little more water to reach your desired consistency.

Transfer the sorbet mixture to a shallow dish or loaf pan and smooth the top with a spatula.

Cover the dish or pan with plastic wrap and place it in the freezer for at least 4 hours or until firm.

Once the sorbet is frozen, scoop it into bowls and garnish with fresh mint leaves if desired.

Calories: 90 | Total Fat: 0.5g | Sodium: 0mg | Potassium: 200mg | Total Carbohydrates: 24g | Dietary Fiber: 3g | Sugars: 16g | Protein: 1g

Almond Cookies

Preparation Time: 15 minutes | Cooking Time: 12 minutes | Serving Size: 12 cookies

Ingredients:

- 1 cup almond flour
- 1/4 cup honey or sweetener of choice
- 1/4 cup unsalted butter, melted
- 1 teaspoon almond extract
- 1/4 teaspoon baking soda
- Pinch of salt

Instructions:

Preheat your oven to 350°F (175°C) and line a baking sheet with parchment paper. In a mixing bowl, combine the almond flour, honey, melted butter, almond extract, baking soda, and salt. Mix until well combined.
Roll the dough into small balls, about 1 inch in diameter, and place them on the prepared baking sheet.
Use a fork to gently flatten each ball of dough, creating a crisscross pattern on top.
Bake in the preheated oven for about 12 minutes or until the cookies are golden brown around the edges.
Remove from the oven and let the cookies cool on the baking sheet for a few minutes before transferring them to a wire rack to cool completely.

Nutrition Facts (per serving):

Calories: 100 | Total Fat: 8g | Sodium: 40mg | Potassium: 10mg | Total Carbohydrates: 6g | Dietary Fiber: 1g | Sugars: 4g | Protein: 2g

Lemon Bars

Preparation Time: 15 minutes | Cooking Time: 25 minutes | Serving Size: 9 bars

Ingredients:

- 1 cup almond flour
- 1/4 cup coconut flour
- 1/4 cup honey or sweetener of choice
- 1/4 cup unsalted butter, melted
- 4 eggs
- 1/2 cup fresh lemon juice
- Zest of 1 lemon
- 1/4 teaspoon baking soda
- Pinch of salt
- Powdered erythritol or powdered sweetener for dusting (optional)

Instructions:

Preheat your oven to 350°F (175°C) and line an 8x8-inch baking dish with parchment paper.

In a mixing bowl, combine the almond flour, coconut flour, honey, melted butter, baking soda, and salt. Mix until well combined.

Press the dough evenly into the bottom of the prepared baking dish.

Bake in the preheated oven for about 12-15 minutes or until the crust is lightly golden brown.

While the crust is baking, prepare the lemon filling. In another mixing bowl, whisk together the eggs, fresh lemon juice, and lemon zest until smooth.

Pour the lemon filling over the baked crust and return to the oven.

Bake for an additional 10-12 minutes or until the filling is set.

Remove from the oven and let the lemon bars cool completely in the baking dish.

Once cooled, slice into bars and dust with powdered erythritol or powdered sweetener if desired.

Calories: 160 | Total Fat: 10g | Sodium: 50mg | Potassium: 50mg | Total Carbohydrates: 12g | Dietary Fiber: 2g | Sugars: 7g | Protein: 4g

Vanilla Rice Pudding

Preparation Time: 5 minutes | Cooking Time: 30 minutes | Serving Size: 4 servings

Ingredients:

- 1/2 cup white rice
- 2 cups milk (dairy or non-dairy)
- 1/4 cup honey or sweetener of choice
- 1 teaspoon vanilla extract
- 1/4 teaspoon ground cinnamon
- Pinch of salt
- Optional toppings: fresh fruit, nuts, or cinnamon

Instructions:

In a saucepan, combine the rice, milk, honey, vanilla extract, ground cinnamon, and salt.
Bring the mixture to a gentle boil over medium heat, then reduce the heat to low.
Simmer the rice pudding uncovered, stirring occasionally, for about 25-30 minutes or until the rice is tender and the mixture has thickened to your desired consistency.
Remove from heat and let the pudding cool slightly before serving.
Serve warm or chilled, optionally topped with fresh fruit, nuts, or a sprinkle of cinnamon.

Nutrition Facts (per serving):

Calories: 200 | Total Fat: 3g | Sodium: 80mg | Potassium: 150mg | Total Carbohydrates: 38g | Dietary Fiber: 0.5g | Sugars: 20g | Protein: 5g

Chocolate Avocado Mousse

Preparation Time: 10 minutes | Cooking Time: 0 minutes | Serving Size: 4 servings

Ingredients:

- 2 ripe avocados
- 1/4 cup unsweetened cocoa powder
- 1/4 cup honey or sweetener of choice
- 1 teaspoon vanilla extract
- Pinch of salt
- Optional toppings: sliced strawberries, shaved chocolate, or whipped cream

Instructions:

Cut the avocados in half, remove the pits, and scoop the flesh into a blender or food processor.

Add the cocoa powder, honey, vanilla extract, and salt to the blender or food processor.

Blend until smooth and creamy, scraping down the sides as needed.

Taste the mousse and adjust the sweetness if necessary by adding more honey.

Divide the mousse among serving dishes.

Chill in the refrigerator for at least 30 minutes before serving.

Garnish with sliced strawberries, shaved chocolate, or a dollop of whipped cream if desired.

Nutrition Facts (per serving):

Calories: 200 | Total Fat: 12g | Sodium: 5mg | Potassium: 470mg | Total Carbohydrates: 25g | Dietary Fiber: 7g | Sugars: 15g | Protein: 3g

Carrot Cake (low sodium, low potassium)

Preparation Time: 20 minutes | Cooking Time: 30 minutes | Serving Size: 12 servings

Ingredients:

- 2 cups grated carrots
- 1/2 cup unsweetened applesauce
- 1/2 cup honey or sweetener of choice
- 1/4 cup vegetable oil
- 2 eggs
- 1 teaspoon vanilla extract
- 1 1/2 cups all-purpose flour
- 1 teaspoon baking powder
- 1/2 teaspoon baking soda
- 1 teaspoon ground cinnamon
- 1/4 teaspoon ground nutmeg
- 1/4 teaspoon ground ginger
- 1/4 cup chopped walnuts (optional)
- Cream cheese frosting (optional)

Instructions:

Preheat your oven to 350°F (175°C) and grease a 9x13-inch baking dish.

In a large mixing bowl, combine the grated carrots, applesauce, honey, vegetable oil, eggs, and vanilla extract. Mix until well combined.

In a separate bowl, sift together the flour, baking powder, baking soda, cinnamon, nutmeg, and ginger.

Gradually add the dry ingredients to the wet ingredients, stirring until just combined. If using, fold in the chopped walnuts.

Pour the batter into the prepared baking dish and spread it out evenly.

Bake in the preheated oven for 25-30 minutes or until a toothpick inserted into the center comes out clean.

Remove from the oven and let the cake cool completely before frosting, if desired.

Calories: 180 | Total Fat: 7g | Sodium: 80mg | Potassium: 120mg | Total Carbohydrates: 28g | Dietary Fiber: 2g | Sugars: 15g | Protein: 3g

Peach Cobbler

Preparation Time: 15 minutes | Cooking Time: 40 minutes | Serving Size: 6 servings

Ingredients:

- 4 cups sliced peaches (fresh or canned in juice, drained)
- 1/4 cup honey or sweetener of choice
- 1 teaspoon vanilla extract
- 1 cup all-purpose flour
- 1/2 cup rolled oats
- 1/4 cup unsalted butter, melted
- 1/4 cup milk (dairy or non-dairy)
- 1 teaspoon baking powder
- 1/4 teaspoon ground cinnamon
- Pinch of salt

Instructions:

Preheat your oven to 375°F (190°C) and grease a 9x9-inch baking dish.

In a mixing bowl, combine the sliced peaches, honey, and vanilla extract. Toss to coat the peaches evenly, then spread them in the prepared baking dish.

In another bowl, mix together the flour, rolled oats, melted butter, milk, baking powder, cinnamon, and salt until well combined.

Drop spoonfuls of the batter over the peaches in the baking dish, spreading it out evenly.

Bake in the preheated oven for about 35-40 minutes or until the topping is golden brown and the peaches are bubbling.

Remove from the oven and let the cobbler cool slightly before serving.

Serve warm, optionally topped with a scoop of vanilla ice cream or a dollop of whipped cream.

Calories: 250 | Total Fat: 8g | Sodium: 90mg | Potassium: 250mg | Total Carbohydrates: 42g | Dietary Fiber: 3g | Sugars: 22g | Protein: 4g

Blueberry Crisp

Preparation Time: 15 minutes | Cooking Time: 40 minutes | Serving Size: 6 servings

Ingredients:

- 4 cups fresh or frozen blueberries
- 1/4 cup honey or sweetener of choice
- 1 tablespoon lemon juice
- 1 teaspoon vanilla extract
- 1 cup old-fashioned oats
- 1/2 cup almond flour
- 1/4 cup chopped nuts (such as almonds or walnuts)
- 1/4 cup unsalted butter, melted
- 1/2 teaspoon ground cinnamon
- Pinch of salt

Instructions:

Preheat your oven to 350°F (175°C) and grease a 9x9-inch baking dish.
In a mixing bowl, combine the blueberries, honey, lemon juice, and vanilla extract.
Toss to coat the blueberries evenly, then spread them in the prepared baking dish.
In another bowl, mix together the oats, almond flour, chopped nuts, melted butter, cinnamon, and salt until well combined.
Sprinkle the oat mixture evenly over the blueberries in the baking dish.
Bake in the preheated oven for about 35-40 minutes or until the topping is golden brown and the blueberries are bubbling.
Remove from the oven and let the crisp cool slightly before serving.
Serve warm, optionally topped with a scoop of vanilla ice cream or a dollop of whipped cream.

Calories: 220 | Total Fat: 10g | Sodium: 5mg | Potassium: 200mg | Total Carbohydrates: 32g | Dietary Fiber: 5g | Sugars: 18g | Protein: 4g

Baked Apples with Cinnamon

Preparation Time: 10 minutes | Cooking Time: 30 minutes | Serving Size: 2 servings

Ingredients:

- 2 apples (such as Granny Smith or Honeycrisp), cored
- 2 tablespoons honey or sweetener of choice
- 1 teaspoon ground cinnamon
- 2 tablespoons chopped nuts (such as walnuts or pecans)
- Optional: a drizzle of maple syrup or a dollop of Greek yogurt for serving

Instructions:

Preheat your oven to 375°F (190°C).

Place the cored apples in a baking dish.

In a small bowl, mix together the honey and cinnamon until well combined.

Spoon the honey-cinnamon mixture into the center of each apple, filling the cavities.

Sprinkle chopped nuts over the top of each apple.

Bake in the preheated oven for about 25-30 minutes or until the apples are tender and slightly caramelized.

Remove from the oven and let the baked apples cool slightly before serving.

Serve warm, optionally drizzled with maple syrup or topped with a dollop of Greek yogurt.

Calories: 150 | Total Fat: 5g | Sodium: 0mg | Potassium: 200mg | Total Carbohydrates: 30g | Dietary Fiber: 4g | Sugars: 24g | Protein: 1g

Strawberry Pie

Preparation Time: 20 minutes | Cooking Time: 0 minutes | Serving Size: 8 servings

Ingredients:

- 1 pre-made pie crust (store-bought or homemade)
- 4 cups fresh strawberries, hulled and sliced
- 1/2 cup honey or sweetener of choice
- 2 tablespoons cornstarch
- 2 tablespoons water
- Optional: whipped cream or vanilla ice cream for serving

Instructions:

If using a pre-made pie crust, follow the package instructions for blind baking. If making a homemade crust, bake it according to the recipe instructions and let it cool completely.

In a saucepan, combine the sliced strawberries and honey over medium heat. Cook for about 5 minutes, stirring occasionally, until the strawberries release their juices.

In a small bowl, mix together the cornstarch and water until smooth. Stir the cornstarch mixture into the strawberries and continue to cook for another 2-3 minutes, or until the mixture has thickened.

Remove the strawberry filling from the heat and let it cool slightly.

Pour the strawberry filling into the cooled pie crust, spreading it out evenly.

Refrigerate the pie for at least 2 hours or until set.

Serve chilled, optionally topped with whipped cream or vanilla ice cream.

Calories: 200 | Total Fat: 7g | Sodium: 90mg | Potassium: 250mg | Total Carbohydrates: 36g | Dietary Fiber: 3g | Sugars: 20g | Protein: 2g

Berry Gelatin

Preparation Time: 5 minutes | Cooking Time: 5 minutes | Serving Size: 4 servings

Ingredients:

- 1 cup mixed berries (such as strawberries, blueberries, raspberries)
- 1 tablespoon honey or sweetener of choice
- 1 tablespoon gelatin powder
- 1 cup water

Instructions:

In a saucepan, combine the mixed berries, honey, and water. Bring to a boil over medium heat.

Once boiling, reduce the heat and let simmer for about 3-4 minutes until the berries start to break down and release their juices.

Remove from heat and stir in the gelatin powder until completely dissolved.

Pour the mixture into serving glasses or molds.

Refrigerate for at least 2 hours or until set.

Serve chilled.

Calories: 30 | Total Fat: 0g | Sodium: 5mg | Potassium: 70mg | Total Carbohydrates: 6g | Dietary Fiber: 1g | Sugars: 4g | Protein: 1g

Vanilla Rice Pudding

Preparation Time: 5 minutes | Cooking Time: 30 minutes | Serving Size: 4 servings

Ingredients:

- 1/2 cup white rice
- 2 cups milk (dairy or non-dairy)
- 1/4 cup honey or sweetener of choice
- 1 teaspoon vanilla extract
- 1/4 teaspoon ground cinnamon
- Pinch of salt

Instructions:

In a saucepan, combine the rice, milk, honey, vanilla extract, cinnamon, and salt.
Bring the mixture to a gentle boil over medium heat, then reduce the heat to low.
Simmer the rice pudding uncovered, stirring occasionally, for about 25-30 minutes or
until the rice is tender and the mixture has thickened to your desired consistency.
Remove from heat and let the pudding cool slightly before serving.
Serve warm or chilled, optionally sprinkled with additional cinnamon on top.

**Calories: 200 | Total Fat: 3g | Sodium: 80mg | Potassium: 150mg | Total
Carbohydrates: 38g | Dietary Fiber: 0.5g | Sugars: 18g | Protein: 3g**

Peach Cobbler

Preparation Time: 15 minutes | Cooking Time: 40 minutes | Serving Size: 6 servings

Ingredients:

- 4 cups sliced peaches (fresh or canned in juice, drained)
- 1/4 cup honey or sweetener of choice
- 1 teaspoon vanilla extract
- 1 cup all-purpose flour
- 1/2 cup rolled oats
- 1/4 cup unsalted butter, melted
- 1/4 cup milk (dairy or non-dairy)
- 1 teaspoon baking powder
- 1/4 teaspoon ground cinnamon
- Pinch of salt

Instructions:

Preheat your oven to 375°F (190°C) and grease a 9x9-inch baking dish.

In a mixing bowl, combine the sliced peaches, honey, and vanilla extract. Toss to coat the peaches evenly, then spread them in the prepared baking dish.

In another bowl, mix together the flour, rolled oats, melted butter, milk, baking powder, cinnamon, and salt until well combined.

Drop spoonfuls of the batter over the peaches in the baking dish, spreading it out evenly.

Bake in the preheated oven for about 35-40 minutes or until the topping is golden brown and the peaches are bubbling.

Remove from the oven and let the cobbler cool slightly before serving.

Serve warm, optionally topped with a scoop of vanilla ice cream or a dollop of whipped cream.

Calories: 250 | Total Fat: 8g | Sodium: 80mg | Potassium: 250mg | Total Carbohydrates: 42g | Dietary Fiber: 3g | Sugars: 22g | Protein: 4g

Special Section: Recipes for Dialysis Patients

For individuals undergoing dialysis, nutrition plays a pivotal role in managing health and enhancing the effectiveness of treatments. Dialysis patients have unique dietary needs, often requiring more protein while needing to carefully manage fluid intake, potassium, phosphorus, and sodium levels. The challenge lies in creating meals that are not only nutritious and supportive of their health needs but also flavorful and enjoyable to eat.

This special section is dedicated to providing recipes specifically tailored for those undergoing dialysis. The focus is on high-quality protein sources to help maintain muscle mass and repair tissues, while also considering the importance of limiting fluids and certain minerals that dialysis does not fully remove from the body. Additionally, these recipes aim to keep sodium intake low to help manage blood pressure and fluid retention, which is a common concern for dialysis patients.

The goal is to offer a variety of recipes that make meals pleasurable and satisfying, without compromising dietary restrictions. Each recipe has been thoughtfully developed to ensure it meets the nutritional guidelines recommended for dialysis patients, helping to alleviate some of the stress associated with meal planning. From hearty breakfasts to nourishing dinners and even tempting snacks and desserts, these recipes provide options to support the dietary needs and enhance the well-being of individuals on dialysis.

Let's explore delicious, kidney-friendly recipes that cater to the specific needs of dialysis patients, ensuring that every meal not only nourishes the body but also delights the palate.

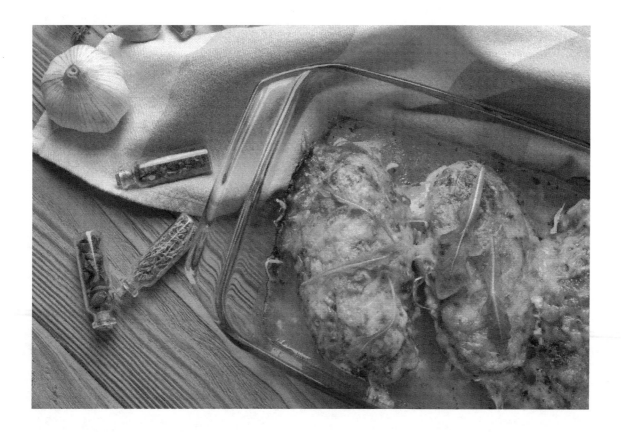

Oven-Baked Chicken Parmesan

Preparation Time: 15 minutes | Cooking Time: 25 minutes | Serving Size: 4 servings

Ingredients:

- 4 boneless, skinless chicken breasts
- 1/2 cup breadcrumbs (preferably low-sodium)
- 1/4 cup grated Parmesan cheese
- 1 teaspoon dried oregano
- 1 teaspoon dried basil
- 1/2 teaspoon garlic powder
- Salt and pepper, to taste
- 1 egg, beaten
- 1 cup marinara sauce (preferably low-sodium)
- 1/2 cup shredded mozzarella cheese
- Fresh basil leaves, for garnish (optional)

Instructions:

Preheat your oven to 400°F (200°C) and line a baking sheet with parchment paper.
In a shallow dish, mix together the breadcrumbs, grated Parmesan cheese, dried oregano, dried basil, garlic powder, salt, and pepper.
Dip each chicken breast into the beaten egg, then coat evenly with the breadcrumb mixture.
Place the coated chicken breasts on the prepared baking sheet.
Bake in the preheated oven for 20 minutes.
Remove the chicken from the oven and spoon marinara sauce over each breast.
Sprinkle shredded mozzarella cheese over the top of each chicken breast.
Return the chicken to the oven and bake for an additional 5 minutes, or until the cheese is melted and bubbly.
Garnish with fresh basil leaves before serving, if desired.

Calories: 300 | Total Fat: 10g | Sodium: 400mg | Potassium: 400mg | Total Carbohydrates: 15g | Dietary Fiber: 2g | Sugars: 3g | Protein: 35g

Eggplant Rollatini

Preparation Time: 20 minutes | Cooking Time: 40 minutes | Serving Size: 4 servings

Ingredients:

- 1 large eggplant, sliced lengthwise into 1/4-inch thick slices
- Salt, for sweating the eggplant
- 1 cup ricotta cheese
- 1/4 cup grated Parmesan cheese
- 1 egg
- 1 teaspoon dried oregano
- 1 teaspoon dried basil
- 1/2 teaspoon garlic powder
- Salt and pepper, to taste
- 1 cup marinara sauce (preferably low-sodium)
- 1/2 cup shredded mozzarella cheese
- Fresh basil leaves, for garnish (optional)

Instructions:

Preheat your oven to 375°F (190°C). Place the eggplant slices on a paper towel-lined baking sheet and sprinkle with salt. Let sit for 15 minutes to draw out excess moisture.

Rinse the eggplant slices under cold water and pat dry with paper towels.

In a mixing bowl, combine the ricotta cheese, grated Parmesan cheese, egg, dried oregano, dried basil, garlic powder, salt, and pepper.

Spread a spoonful of the ricotta mixture onto each eggplant slice, then roll up tightly. Place the rolled eggplant slices seam-side down in a baking dish.

Pour marinara sauce over the rolled eggplant slices, then sprinkle shredded mozzarella cheese on top.

Cover the baking dish with foil and bake in the preheated oven for 30 minutes.

Remove the foil and bake for an additional 10 minutes, or until the cheese is melted and bubbly.

Garnish with fresh basil leaves before serving, if desired.

Calories: 250 | Total Fat: 12g | Sodium: 350mg | Potassium: 400mg | Total Carbohydrates: 15g | Dietary Fiber: 5g | Sugars: 7g | Protein: 15g

Grilled Vegetable Platter with Lemon-Herb Drizzle

Preparation Time: 15 minutes | Cooking Time: 15 minutes | Serving Size: 4 servings

Ingredients:

- 2 zucchinis, sliced lengthwise
- 2 yellow squash, sliced lengthwise
- 1 red bell pepper, seeded and quartered
- 1 yellow bell pepper, seeded and quartered
- 1 red onion, sliced into thick rounds
- 1 tablespoon olive oil
- Salt and pepper, to taste
- Fresh herbs (such as parsley, basil, or thyme), for garnish
- Lemon-Herb Drizzle:
  - 2 tablespoons olive oil
  - 1 tablespoon fresh lemon juice
  - 1 garlic clove, minced
  - 1 teaspoon dried oregano
  - 1 teaspoon dried thyme
  - Salt and pepper, to taste

Instructions:

Preheat your grill to medium-high heat.

In a small bowl, whisk together the ingredients for the Lemon-Herb Drizzle: olive oil, lemon juice, minced garlic, dried oregano, dried thyme, salt, and pepper. Set aside.

Brush the zucchini, yellow squash, bell peppers, and red onion slices with olive oil and season with salt and pepper.

Place the vegetables on the preheated grill and cook for about 4-5 minutes per side, or until grill marks appear and the vegetables are tender.

Arrange the grilled vegetables on a serving platter.

Drizzle the Lemon-Herb Drizzle over the grilled vegetables.

Garnish with fresh herbs before serving.

Calories: 120 | Total Fat: 8g | Sodium: 20mg | Potassium: 350mg | Total Carbohydrates: 10g | Dietary Fiber: 3g | Sugars: 5g | Protein: 2g

Turkey and Sweet Potato Shepherd's Pie

Preparation Time: 20 minutes | Cooking Time: 40 minutes | Serving Size: 6 servings

Ingredients:

- 1 pound ground turkey
- 1 onion, chopped
- 2 cloves garlic, minced
- 2 cups diced carrots
- 1 cup frozen peas
- 1 cup low-sodium chicken broth
- 2 tablespoons tomato paste
- 1 teaspoon dried thyme
- Salt and pepper, to taste
- 3 large sweet potatoes, peeled and diced
- 2 tablespoons unsalted butter
- 1/4 cup milk (dairy or non-dairy)
- Fresh parsley, chopped, for garnish

Instructions:

Preheat your oven to 375°F (190°C).

In a large skillet, cook the ground turkey over medium heat until browned. Drain any excess fat.

Add the chopped onion and minced garlic to the skillet with the turkey. Cook for 2-3 minutes until the onion is translucent.

Stir in the diced carrots, frozen peas, chicken broth, tomato paste, dried thyme, salt, and pepper. Simmer for 10-15 minutes until the vegetables are tender and the mixture has thickened.

While the turkey mixture is simmering, place the diced sweet potatoes in a pot of water. Bring to a boil and cook until the sweet potatoes are fork-tender, about 15 minutes.

Drain the sweet potatoes and transfer them to a mixing bowl. Add the butter and milk, then mash until smooth.

Transfer the turkey mixture to a baking dish. Spread the mashed sweet potatoes over the top.

Bake in the preheated oven for 20-25 minutes, or until the top is lightly browned and the filling is bubbly.

Garnish with chopped fresh parsley before serving.

Calories: 300 | Total Fat: 10g | Sodium: 200mg | Potassium: 450mg | Total Carbohydrates: 30g | Dietary Fiber: 5g | Sugars: 8g | Protein: 20g

Beef Sloppy Joes (low sodium)

Preparation Time: 10 minutes | Cooking Time: 20 minutes | Serving Size: 4 servings

Ingredients:

- 1 pound lean ground beef
- 1 onion, chopped
- 1 green bell pepper, chopped
- 2 cloves garlic, minced
- 1 cup low-sodium tomato sauce
- 2 tablespoons tomato paste
- 1 tablespoon Worcestershire sauce (low sodium)
- 1 tablespoon apple cider vinegar
- 1 tablespoon brown sugar
- 1 teaspoon mustard powder
- Salt and pepper, to taste
- Whole grain hamburger buns, for serving

Instructions:

In a large skillet, cook the ground beef over medium heat until browned.

Add the chopped onion, green bell pepper, and minced garlic to the skillet. Cook for 5 minutes, or until the vegetables are softened.

Stir in the tomato sauce, tomato paste, Worcestershire sauce, apple cider vinegar, brown sugar, mustard powder, salt, and pepper. Simmer for 10 minutes, stirring occasionally, until the sauce thickens.

Serve the beef mixture on whole grain hamburger buns.

Calories: 300 | Total Fat: 12g | Sodium: 200mg | Potassium: 350mg | Total Carbohydrates: 20g | Dietary Fiber: 3g | Sugars: 7g | Protein: 25g

Low-Potassium Potato Salad

Preparation Time: 15 minutes | Cooking Time: 20 minutes | Serving Size: 4 servings

Ingredients:

- 1 pound red potatoes, diced
- 1/2 cup plain Greek yogurt (low-fat or fat-free)
- 2 tablespoons lemon juice
- 1 tablespoon Dijon mustard
- 1 tablespoon chopped fresh dill
- 2 green onions, thinly sliced
- Salt and pepper, to taste
- Optional: chopped celery, chopped parsley, diced cucumber

Instructions:

Place the diced potatoes in a pot and cover with water. Bring to a boil, then reduce heat and simmer for 15-20 minutes until the potatoes are fork-tender.

Drain the cooked potatoes and let them cool slightly.

In a large mixing bowl, whisk together the Greek yogurt, lemon juice, Dijon mustard, chopped dill, green onions, salt, and pepper.

Add the cooked potatoes to the bowl and toss to coat evenly with the dressing.

Optional: Add chopped celery, parsley, or diced cucumber for extra flavor and texture.

Serve the potato salad immediately, or refrigerate for a few hours to chill before serving.

Calories: 150 | Total Fat: 0.5g | Sodium: 100mg | Potassium: 300mg | Total Carbohydrates: 30g | Dietary Fiber: 3g | Sugars: 2g | Protein: 5g

Cranberry Almond Energy Bites

Preparation Time: 10 minutes | Cooking Time: 0 minutes | Serving Size: 12 bites

Ingredients:

- 1 cup old-fashioned oats
- 1/2 cup almond butter
- 1/4 cup honey
- 1/4 cup dried cranberries
- 1/4 cup chopped almonds
- 1 tablespoon chia seeds
- 1 teaspoon vanilla extract
- Pinch of salt

Instructions:

In a mixing bowl, combine all ingredients: oats, almond butter, honey, dried cranberries, chopped almonds, chia seeds, vanilla extract, and a pinch of salt.
Stir until well combined and the mixture is sticky.
Roll the mixture into small balls, about 1 inch in diameter, and place them on a baking sheet lined with parchment paper.
Place the baking sheet in the refrigerator for at least 30 minutes to firm up the energy bites.
Once firm, transfer the energy bites to an airtight container and store them in the refrigerator for up to one week.

Calories: 120 | Total Fat: 6g | Sodium: 20mg | Potassium: 100mg | Total Carbohydrates: 15g | Dietary Fiber: 2g | Sugars: 8g | Protein: 3g

Zesty Lime Shrimp and Avocado Salad

Preparation Time: 15 minutes | Cooking Time: 5 minutes | Serving Size: 4 servings

Ingredients:

- 1 pound large shrimp, peeled and deveined
- 2 avocados, diced
- 1 cup cherry tomatoes, halved
- 1/4 cup red onion, thinly sliced
- 1/4 cup fresh cilantro, chopped
- 2 tablespoons olive oil
- 2 tablespoons lime juice
- 1 teaspoon honey (optional)
- Salt and pepper, to taste
- Optional: jalapeño slices for added spice

Instructions:

Heat olive oil in a skillet over medium-high heat.
Season shrimp with salt and pepper, then add them to the skillet.
Cook shrimp for 2-3 minutes on each side until they are pink and opaque.
In a large mixing bowl, combine diced avocado, cherry tomatoes, sliced red onion, and chopped cilantro.
In a small bowl, whisk together lime juice and honey (if using).
Pour the lime dressing over the avocado mixture and toss gently to coat.
Add cooked shrimp to the bowl and toss to combine.
Serve immediately, garnished with additional cilantro and jalapeño slices if desired.

Calories: 250 | Total Fat: 15g | Sodium: 200mg | Potassium: 600mg | Total Carbohydrates: 12g | Dietary Fiber: 6g | Sugars: 4g | Protein: 20g

Sautéed Garlic Spinach

Preparation Time: 5 minutes | Cooking Time: 5 minutes | Serving Size: 4 servings

Ingredients:

- 1 tablespoon olive oil
- 2 cloves garlic, minced
- 1 pound fresh spinach leaves, washed and drained
- Salt and pepper, to taste
- Optional: red pepper flakes for added heat

Instructions:

Heat olive oil in a large skillet over medium heat.

Add minced garlic to the skillet and cook for about 1 minute until fragrant.

Add the fresh spinach leaves to the skillet. Use tongs to toss the spinach in the garlic and oil until wilted, about 2-3 minutes.

Season with salt, pepper, and red pepper flakes if desired.

Once the spinach is wilted and tender, remove from heat.

Serve immediately as a side dish or as part of a main course.

Calories: 50 | Total Fat: 3g | Sodium: 100mg | Potassium: 600mg | Total Carbohydrates: 5g | Dietary Fiber: 3g | Sugars: 0g | Protein: 3g

High-Protein Chicken Salad

Preparation Time: 15 minutes | Cooking Time: 20 minutes | Serving Size: 4 servings

Ingredients:

- 2 boneless, skinless chicken breasts
- 1/4 cup plain Greek yogurt
- 2 tablespoons mayonnaise (low-fat or fat-free)
- 1 tablespoon Dijon mustard
- 1 stalk celery, diced
- 1/4 cup red onion, finely chopped
- 1/4 cup grapes, halved
- 1/4 cup chopped walnuts
- Salt and pepper, to taste
- Optional: lettuce leaves, for serving

Instructions:

In a pot, bring water to a boil. Add chicken breasts and cook for 15-20 minutes until fully cooked.

Remove chicken from water and let it cool. Once cooled, shred the chicken into bite-sized pieces.

In a mixing bowl, combine the shredded chicken, Greek yogurt, mayonnaise, and Dijon mustard. Mix well.

Add diced celery, chopped red onion, halved grapes, and chopped walnuts to the bowl. Stir until all ingredients are evenly coated.

Season with salt and pepper to taste.

Serve the chicken salad on lettuce leaves for a low-carb option, or enjoy it on whole grain bread or crackers.

Calories: 250 | Total Fat: 12g | Sodium: 200mg | Potassium: 300mg | Total Carbohydrates: 5g | Dietary Fiber: 2g | Sugars: 3g | Protein: 25g

Salmon Patties with Dill Sauce

Preparation Time: 15 minutes | Cooking Time: 10 minutes | Serving Size: 4 servings

Ingredients:

- 2 cans (6 ounces each) salmon, drained and flaked
- 1/4 cup breadcrumbs (preferably low-sodium)
- 1/4 cup finely chopped onion
- 2 tablespoons chopped fresh parsley
- 1 egg, beaten
- 1 tablespoon lemon juice
- 1 teaspoon Dijon mustard
- Salt and pepper, to taste
- 1 tablespoon olive oil

Dill Sauce:

- 1/2 cup plain Greek yogurt
- 1 tablespoon chopped fresh dill
- 1 teaspoon lemon juice
- Salt and pepper, to taste

Instructions:

In a large mixing bowl, combine the flaked salmon, breadcrumbs, chopped onion, chopped parsley, beaten egg, lemon juice, Dijon mustard, salt, and pepper. Mix until well combined.

Divide the mixture into 4 equal portions and shape each portion into a patty.

Heat olive oil in a skillet over medium heat. Add the salmon patties and cook for 3-4 minutes on each side until golden brown and cooked through.

While the patties are cooking, prepare the dill sauce. In a small bowl, combine the Greek yogurt, chopped dill, lemon juice, salt, and pepper. Mix well.

Serve the salmon patties hot with a dollop of dill sauce on top.

Calories: 250 | Total Fat: 12g | Sodium: 300mg | Potassium: 400mg | Total Carbohydrates: 10g | Dietary Fiber: 2g | Sugars: 2g | Protein: 25g

Roasted Turkey Breast with Green Beans

Preparation Time: 15 minutes | Cooking Time: 1 hour | Serving Size: 4 servings

Ingredients:

- 1 turkey breast (about 2 pounds), bone-in and skin-on
- 1 pound fresh green beans, trimmed
- 2 tablespoons olive oil
- 2 cloves garlic, minced
- 1 teaspoon dried thyme
- 1 teaspoon dried rosemary
- Salt and pepper, to taste

Instructions:

Preheat your oven to 375°F (190°C).

Place the turkey breast in a roasting pan, skin side up.

In a small bowl, mix together olive oil, minced garlic, dried thyme, dried rosemary, salt, and pepper.

Rub the olive oil mixture over the turkey breast, making sure it is evenly coated.

Arrange the green beans around the turkey breast in the roasting pan.

Roast in the preheated oven for about 1 hour, or until the turkey breast reaches an internal temperature of 165°F (74°C) and the juices run clear.

Once cooked, remove the turkey breast from the oven and let it rest for a few minutes before slicing.

Serve the roasted turkey breast with green beans on the side.

Nutrition Facts (per serving):

Calories: 300 | Total Fat: 10g | Sodium: 200mg | Potassium: 450mg | Total Carbohydrates: 10g | Dietary Fiber: 4g | Sugars: 3g | Protein: 40g

Pork Tenderloin with Applesauce

Preparation Time: 10 minutes | Cooking Time: 25 minutes | Serving Size: 4 servings

Ingredients:

- 1 pork tenderloin (about 1 pound)
- 2 tablespoons olive oil
- 1 teaspoon dried thyme
- 1 teaspoon dried rosemary
- Salt and pepper, to taste

Applesauce:

- 2 apples, peeled, cored, and diced
- 1/4 cup water
- 1 tablespoon honey (optional)
- 1/2 teaspoon ground cinnamon

Instructions:

Preheat your oven to 400°F (200°C).

Season the pork tenderloin with dried thyme, dried rosemary, salt, and pepper.

Heat olive oil in an ovenproof skillet over medium-high heat. Add the pork tenderloin and sear on all sides until browned, about 2-3 minutes per side.

Transfer the skillet to the preheated oven and roast for about 20 minutes, or until the internal temperature of the pork reaches 145°F (63°C).

While the pork is cooking, prepare the applesauce. In a saucepan, combine diced apples, water, honey (if using), and ground cinnamon. Cook over medium heat until the apples are soft and tender, about 10-15 minutes. Mash the apples with a fork or potato masher to desired consistency.

Once the pork is cooked through, remove it from the oven and let it rest for a few minutes before slicing.

Serve the sliced pork tenderloin with a dollop of applesauce on top.

Calories: 250 | Total Fat: 10g | Sodium: 100mg | Potassium: 400mg | Total Carbohydrates: 15g | Dietary Fiber: 3g | Sugars: 10g | Protein: 25g

Beef Stew (Modified for Renal Diet)

Preparation Time: 20 minutes | Cooking Time: 2 hours | Serving Size: 6 servings

Ingredients:

- 1 pound beef stew meat, cut into bite-sized pieces
- 1 tablespoon olive oil
- 2 cloves garlic, minced
- 1 onion, chopped
- 2 carrots, sliced
- 2 celery stalks, sliced
- 2 cups low-sodium beef broth
- 1 cup water
- 2 potatoes, peeled and diced
- 1 bay leaf
- Salt and pepper, to taste
- 2 tablespoons chopped fresh parsley, for garnish (optional)

Instructions:

Heat olive oil in a large pot over medium heat. Add the beef stew meat and cook until browned on all sides, about 5 minutes.

Add minced garlic and chopped onion to the pot, and sauté until fragrant, about 2 minutes.

Stir in sliced carrots and celery, and cook for another 5 minutes.

Pour in low-sodium beef broth and water. Bring to a boil, then reduce heat to low.

Add diced potatoes and bay leaf to the pot. Cover and simmer for 1.5 to 2 hours, or until the beef is tender and the vegetables are cooked through.

Season with salt and pepper to taste.

Discard the bay leaf before serving.

Garnish with chopped fresh parsley if desired.

Serve hot and enjoy!

Calories: 250 | Total Fat: 10g | Sodium: 200mg | Potassium: 500mg | Total Carbohydrates: 15g | Dietary Fiber: 3g | Sugars: 3g | Protein: 25g

Grilled Shrimp with Quinoa

Preparation Time: 15 minutes | Cooking Time: 15 minutes | Serving Size: 4 servings

Ingredients:

- 1 pound large shrimp, peeled and deveined
- 1 cup quinoa, rinsed
- 2 cups low-sodium vegetable broth
- 1 tablespoon olive oil
- 2 cloves garlic, minced
- 1 teaspoon smoked paprika
- Salt and pepper, to taste
- Lemon wedges, for serving

Instructions:

In a saucepan, bring the vegetable broth to a boil. Add the quinoa, reduce heat to low, cover, and simmer for 12-15 minutes, or until quinoa is tender and liquid is absorbed. Remove from heat and let it sit, covered, for 5 minutes. Fluff with a fork. Meanwhile, preheat the grill to medium-high heat.

In a bowl, combine the shrimp, olive oil, minced garlic, smoked paprika, salt, and pepper. Toss until the shrimp are evenly coated.

Thread the shrimp onto skewers, then grill for 2-3 minutes on each side until they are pink and opaque.

Serve the grilled shrimp over cooked quinoa, garnished with lemon wedges.

Enjoy hot!

Calories: 300 | Total Fat: 7g | Sodium: 200mg | Potassium: 400mg | Total Carbohydrates: 32g | Dietary Fiber: 4g | Sugars: 1g | Protein: 25g

Baked Sweet Potato Fries

Preparation Time: 10 minutes | Cooking Time: 25 minutes | Serving Size: 4 servings

Ingredients:

- 2 large sweet potatoes, scrubbed and cut into fries
- 2 tablespoons olive oil
- 1 teaspoon garlic powder
- 1 teaspoon paprika
- Salt and pepper, to taste
- Optional: chopped fresh parsley, for garnish

Instructions:

Preheat your oven to 425°F (220°C) and line a baking sheet with parchment paper.
In a large bowl, toss the sweet potato fries with olive oil, garlic powder, paprika, salt, and pepper until evenly coated.
Arrange the fries in a single layer on the prepared baking sheet, making sure they are not overcrowded.
Bake in the preheated oven for 20-25 minutes, flipping halfway through, until the fries are golden brown and crispy.
Once done, remove from the oven and let them cool slightly before serving.
Garnish with chopped fresh parsley, if desired.
Serve hot and enjoy!

Calories: 150 | Total Fat: 7g | Sodium: 100mg | Potassium: 300mg | Total Carbohydrates: 20g | Dietary Fiber: 3g | Sugars: 5g | Protein: 2g

Chicken Noodle Soup (Low Potassium, Low Phosphorus)

Preparation Time: 15 minutes | Cooking Time: 30 minutes | Serving Size: 6 servings

Ingredients:

- 1 tablespoon olive oil
- 1 onion, diced
- 2 carrots, sliced
- 2 celery stalks, sliced
- 2 cloves garlic, minced
- 6 cups low-sodium chicken broth
- 2 cups water
- 2 boneless, skinless chicken breasts, cooked and shredded
- 2 cups uncooked egg noodles
- 1 teaspoon dried thyme
- Salt and pepper, to taste
- Chopped fresh parsley, for garnish (optional)

Instructions:

In a large pot, heat olive oil over medium heat. Add diced onion, sliced carrots, and sliced celery. Cook until vegetables are softened, about 5 minutes.
Add minced garlic and cook for an additional 1-2 minutes until fragrant.
Pour in low-sodium chicken broth and water. Bring to a boil.
Once boiling, add shredded chicken, uncooked egg noodles, and dried thyme to the pot. Reduce heat to medium-low and simmer for 10-12 minutes, or until noodles are cooked through.
Season with salt and pepper to taste.
Serve hot, garnished with chopped fresh parsley if desired.

Calories: 200 | Total Fat: 5g | Sodium: 150mg | Potassium: 180mg | Total Carbohydrates: 15g | Dietary Fiber: 2g | Sugars: 3g | Protein: 20g

Egg Salad on Low-Sodium Bread

Preparation Time: 10 minutes | Serving Size: 4 servings

Ingredients:

- 6 hard-boiled eggs, chopped
- 1/4 cup low-fat mayonnaise
- 1 tablespoon Dijon mustard
- 2 tablespoons chopped chives or green onions
- Salt and pepper, to taste
- 8 slices low-sodium bread
- Lettuce leaves, for serving (optional)
- Tomato slices, for serving (optional)

Instructions:

In a mixing bowl, combine the chopped hard-boiled eggs, low-fat mayonnaise, Dijon mustard, chopped chives or green onions, salt, and pepper. Mix until well combined.
Toast the low-sodium bread slices, if desired.
Spread the egg salad mixture evenly onto 4 slices of bread.
Top with lettuce leaves and tomato slices, if using.
Place the remaining bread slices on top to make sandwiches.
Serve immediately, or wrap tightly and refrigerate for later.

Calories: 250 | Total Fat: 12g | Sodium: 200mg | Potassium: 150mg | Total Carbohydrates: 20g | Dietary Fiber: 3g | Sugars: 2g | Protein: 15g

Dialysis-Friendly Stuffed Peppers

Preparation Time: 15 minutes | Cooking Time: 45 minutes | Serving Size: 4 servings

Ingredients:

- 4 large bell peppers, any color
- 1 cup cooked brown rice (preferably low sodium)
- 1/2 pound lean ground turkey or chicken
- 1 small onion, chopped
- 2 cloves garlic, minced
- 1 cup low-sodium tomato sauce
- 1 teaspoon dried oregano
- 1 teaspoon dried basil
- Salt and pepper, to taste
- 1/4 cup shredded low-sodium mozzarella cheese (optional)
- Fresh parsley, chopped, for garnish (optional)

Instructions:

Preheat your oven to 375°F (190°C).

Cut the tops off the bell peppers and remove the seeds and membranes.

In a skillet, cook the ground turkey or chicken over medium heat until browned.

Add the chopped onion and minced garlic to the skillet with the turkey or chicken. Cook for 2-3 minutes until the onion is translucent.

Stir in the cooked brown rice, tomato sauce, dried oregano, dried basil, salt, and pepper. Cook for another 5 minutes until heated through.

Stuff the bell peppers with the turkey or chicken and rice mixture.

Place the stuffed peppers in a baking dish and cover with foil.

Bake in the preheated oven for 30 minutes.

Remove the foil, sprinkle shredded mozzarella cheese on top of each pepper (if using), and bake for an additional 10-15 minutes until the cheese is melted and bubbly.

Garnish with chopped fresh parsley before serving, if desired.

Calories: 250 | Total Fat: 6g | Sodium: 200mg | Potassium: 500mg | Total Carbohydrates: 30g | Dietary Fiber: 5g | Sugars: 5g | Protein: 20g

High-Protein Smoothie

Preparation Time: 5 minutes | Cooking Time: 0 minutes | Serving Size: 1 serving

Ingredients:

- 1/2 cup plain Greek yogurt
- 1/2 cup unsweetened almond milk (or any milk of choice)
- 1/2 banana, frozen
- 1/2 cup frozen mixed berries (such as strawberries, blueberries, raspberries)
- 1 tablespoon almond butter (or peanut butter)
- 1 tablespoon chia seeds or flaxseeds
- Optional: honey or sweetener of choice, to taste

Instructions:

In a blender, combine the plain Greek yogurt, almond milk, frozen banana, frozen mixed berries, almond butter, and chia seeds.
Blend until smooth and creamy, adding honey or sweetener if desired for extra sweetness.
Pour the smoothie into a glass and enjoy immediately.

Calories: 300 | Total Fat: 12g | Sodium: 100mg | Potassium: 400mg | Total Carbohydrates: 30g | Dietary Fiber: 8g | Sugars: 15g | Protein: 20g

Egg Salad

Preparation Time: 10 minutes | Cooking Time: 10 minutes | Serving Size: 4 servings

Ingredients:

- 6 hard-boiled eggs, peeled and chopped
- 2 tablespoons plain Greek yogurt (low-fat or fat-free)
- 1 tablespoon mayonnaise (low-fat or fat-free)
- 1 teaspoon Dijon mustard
- 1 celery stalk, finely chopped
- 1 green onion, thinly sliced
- Salt and pepper, to taste
- Optional: chopped fresh parsley or chives, for garnish

Instructions:

In a mixing bowl, combine the chopped hard-boiled eggs, plain Greek yogurt, mayonnaise, Dijon mustard, chopped celery, and sliced green onion.
Mix well until all ingredients are evenly combined.
Season with salt and pepper to taste.
Garnish with chopped fresh parsley or chives, if desired.
Serve the egg salad on whole grain bread, lettuce wraps, or enjoy it on its own.

Calories: 150 | Total Fat: 10g | Sodium: 200mg | Potassium: 150mg | Total Carbohydrates: 2g | Dietary Fiber: 0.5g | Sugars: 1g | Protein: 12g

Dialysis-Friendly Stuffed Peppers

Preparation Time: 15 minutes | Cooking Time: 45 minutes | Serving Size: 4 servings

Ingredients:

- 4 large bell peppers, any color
- 1 cup cooked brown rice (preferably low sodium)
- 1/2 pound lean ground turkey or chicken
- 1 small onion, chopped
- 2 cloves garlic, minced
- 1 cup low-sodium tomato sauce
- 1 teaspoon dried oregano
- 1 teaspoon dried basil
- Salt and pepper, to taste
- 1/4 cup shredded low-sodium mozzarella cheese (optional)
- Fresh parsley, chopped, for garnish (optional)

Instructions:

Preheat your oven to 375°F (190°C).
Cut the tops off the bell peppers and remove the seeds and membranes.
In a skillet, cook the ground turkey or chicken over medium heat until browned.
Add the chopped onion and minced garlic to the skillet with the turkey or chicken.
Cook for 2-3 minutes until the onion is translucent.
Stir in the cooked brown rice, tomato sauce, dried oregano, dried basil, salt, and pepper. Cook for another 5 minutes until heated through.
Stuff the bell peppers with the turkey or chicken and rice mixture.
Place the stuffed peppers in a baking dish and cover with foil.
Bake in the preheated oven for 30 minutes.
Remove the foil, sprinkle shredded mozzarella cheese on top of each pepper (if using), and bake for an additional 10-15 minutes until the cheese is melted and bubbly.
Garnish with chopped fresh parsley before serving, if desired.

Calories: 250 | Total Fat: 6g | Sodium: 200mg | Potassium: 500mg | Total Carbohydrates: 30g | Dietary Fiber: 5g | Sugars: 5g | Protein: 20g

High-Protein Smoothie

Preparation Time: 5 minutes | Cooking Time: 0 minutes | Serving Size: 1 serving

Ingredients:

- 1/2 cup plain Greek yogurt
- 1/2 cup unsweetened almond milk (or any milk of choice)
- 1/2 banana, frozen
- 1/2 cup frozen mixed berries (such as strawberries, blueberries, raspberries)
- 1 tablespoon almond butter (or peanut butter)
- 1 tablespoon chia seeds or flaxseeds
- Optional: honey or sweetener of choice, to taste

Instructions:

In a blender, combine the plain Greek yogurt, almond milk, frozen banana, frozen mixed berries, almond butter, and chia seeds.

Blend until smooth and creamy, adding honey or sweetener if desired for extra sweetness.

Pour the smoothie into a glass and enjoy immediately.

Calories: 300 | Total Fat: 12g | Sodium: 100mg | Potassium: 400mg | Total Carbohydrates: 30g | Dietary Fiber: 8g | Sugars: 15g | Protein: 20g

5. 4-Week Meal Plan

Weekly Meal Plans

Week 1

Monday:

- Breakfast: Apple and Cinnamon Porridge
- Lunch: Quinoa Salad with Lemon Vinaigrette
- Dinner: Baked Salmon with Herb Crust; Steamed Broccoli

Tuesday:

- Breakfast: Vanilla Almond Oatmeal
- Lunch: Mediterranean-inspired Stuffed Peppers
- Dinner: Garlic Roasted Cauliflower; Grilled Chicken Wrap

Wednesday:

- Breakfast: Berry Smoothie Bowl
- Lunch: Chicken and Rice Soup
- Dinner: Vegetarian Chili; Side of Cornbread (adapt recipe to be renal-friendly)

Thursday:

- Breakfast: Zucchini and Carrot Muffins
- Lunch: Turkey and Avocado Wrap
- Dinner: Lemon Herb Baked Tilapia with Zucchini Ribbons

Friday:

- Breakfast: Greek Yogurt with Honey and Walnuts
- Lunch: Roasted Beet and Goat Cheese Salad
- Dinner: Stir-Fried Beef and Broccoli

Saturday:

- Breakfast: Savory Mushroom Toast
- Lunch: Avocado Chicken Salad
- Dinner: Pumpkin Pie with Whipped Cream for dessert; Dinner of Lemon Garlic Halibut

Sunday:

- Breakfast: Vegetable Breakfast Burritos
- Lunch: Caprese Salad with Balsamic Glaze
- Dinner: Italian Beef Stew

Week 2

Monday:

- Breakfast: Egg White and Spinach Frittata
- Lunch: Pasta Primavera with Garlic Olive Oil Sauce
- Dinner: Grilled Pork Chops with Apple Slaw

Tuesday:

- Breakfast: Buckwheat Pancakes
- Lunch: Cucumber Tomato Salad with Feta
- Dinner: Turkey Meatballs in Tomato Sauce

Wednesday:

- Breakfast: Renal-Friendly Pancakes
- Lunch: Lentil Soup with Carrots and Celery
- Dinner: Moroccan Tagine with Vegetables

Thursday:

- Breakfast: Low Sodium Omelet
- Lunch: Balsamic Grilled Vegetables
- Dinner: Shrimp Scampi with Zoodles

Friday:

- Breakfast: Vanilla Rice Pudding
- Lunch: Quiche with Egg Whites and Vegetables
- Dinner: Baked Tilapia with Mango Salsa

Saturday:

- Breakfast: Apple Cinnamon Muffins
- Lunch: Tabbouleh with Quinoa
- Dinner: Pork Loin with Apple Compote

Sunday:

- Breakfast: Vegetable Breakfast Burritos (repeat)
- Lunch: Roasted Turkey and Cranberry Wrap
- Dinner: Ratatouille; Dessert of Raspberry Gelatin

Week 3

Monday:

- Breakfast: Apple and Cinnamon Porridge
- Lunch: Quinoa Salad with Lemon Vinaigrette
- Dinner: Baked Salmon with Herb Crust and a side of Garlic Roasted Cauliflower

Tuesday:

- Breakfast: Vanilla Almond Oatmeal
- Lunch: Roasted Turkey and Cranberry Wrap
- Dinner: Vegetarian Stuffed Acorn Squash

Wednesday:

- Breakfast: Berry Smoothie Bowl
- Lunch: Mediterranean-inspired Stuffed Peppers
- Dinner: Lemon Garlic Halibut with Parmesan Roasted Asparagus

Thursday:

- Breakfast: Zucchini and Carrot Muffins
- Lunch: Spinach and Goat Cheese Stuffed Chicken Breast with Cucumber Tomato Salad with Feta
- Dinner: Beef and Vegetable Kabobs

Friday:

- Breakfast: Buckwheat Pancakes
- Lunch: Chicken and Rice Soup
- Dinner: Shrimp Scampi with Zoodles

Saturday:

- Breakfast: Greek Yogurt with Honey and Walnuts
- Lunch: Avocado Chicken Salad
- Dinner: Moroccan Tagine with Vegetables

Sunday:

- Breakfast: Vegetable Breakfast Burritos
- Lunch: Balsamic Grilled Vegetables with a side of Low-Potassium Potato Salad
- Dinner: Maple Glazed Salmon with a side of Broccoli and Carrot Slaw

Week 4

Monday:

- Breakfast: Egg White and Spinach Frittata
- Lunch: Quiche with Egg Whites and Vegetables
- Dinner: Italian Beef Stew with a side of Baked Garlic Parmesan Zucchini Chips

Tuesday:

- Breakfast: Low Sodium Omelet
- Lunch: Grilled Chicken Caesar Salad (Low-Sodium Dressing)
- Dinner: Baked Cod with Parsley Pesto and Radish and Cucumber Salad

Wednesday:

- Breakfast: Savory Mushroom Toast
- Lunch: Asian-inspired Tofu and Sauteed Vegetables
- Dinner: Turkey Meatballs in Tomato Sauce with Edamame Salad

Thursday:

- Breakfast: Renal-Friendly Pancakes
- Lunch: Pasta Primavera with Garlic Olive Oil Sauce
- Dinner: Garlic Lemon Chicken Kebabs with Pineapple Cucumber Salad

Friday:

- Breakfast: Apple Cinnamon Muffins
- Lunch: Lentil Soup with Carrots and Celery
- Dinner: Pork Loin with Apple Compote and a side of Sweet Potato Hash

Saturday:

- Breakfast: Berry Smoothie Bowl (Repeat)
- Lunch: Tabbouleh with Quinoa
- Dinner: Ratatouille with a side of Cheesy Cauliflower Bake

Sunday:

- Breakfast: Greek Yogurt with Honey and Walnuts (Repeat)
- Lunch: Vegetable Soup
- Dinner: Baked Tilapia with Mango Salsa and a side of Stuffed Bell Peppers with Rice and Herbs

Adjusting Meal Plans

Meal plans are essential for managing health, saving time, and reducing food waste. However, individual dietary restrictions, health conditions, or personal preferences can necessitate adjustments. Here's a guide on how to tailor meal plans effectively:

1. Understand Dietary Needs:

- Medical Conditions: Conditions like diabetes, kidney disease, or allergies require specific dietary adjustments. Understanding what nutrients need to be controlled (e.g., sodium, potassium, phosphorus) is crucial.
- Preferences and Restrictions: Whether due to personal preference, religious reasons, or ethical concerns, dietary restrictions vary widely, from vegetarianism to gluten-free diets.

2. Substituting Ingredients:

- Allergies and Intolerances: Substitute allergens with safe alternatives (e.g., almond milk for cow's milk, gluten-free flour for wheat flour).
- Vegetarian or Vegan Diets: Replace animal proteins with plant-based proteins (beans, lentils, tofu). Use nutritional yeast or plant-based cheeses for a cheesy flavor without dairy.
- Low-Sodium, Low-Potassium, Low-Phosphorus Needs: Opt for fresh, unprocessed foods, as they naturally contain less sodium, potassium, and phosphorus than their processed counterparts. Herbs and spices can replace salt for flavor.

3. Portion Control:

Adjust portion sizes based on individual energy needs. This can vary with age, gender, activity level, and specific health goals like weight loss or muscle gain.

4. Planning for Preferences:

- Cultural Preferences: Incorporate traditional foods and flavors into the meal plan to maintain cultural relevance and enjoyment.
- Taste Preferences: If certain spices or ingredients are disliked, find alternatives that satisfy taste buds while maintaining nutritional balance.

5. Reading Labels:

For those managing chronic conditions, reading nutrition labels is vital to avoid hidden sources of restricted nutrients like sodium in canned goods or phosphorus in preservatives.

6. Consult with Professionals:

When adjusting meal plans for health conditions, consult with a healthcare provider or dietitian. They can offer personalized advice that considers medical history, current health status, and nutritional needs.

7. Experiment and Educate:

Learning to cook with new ingredients or trying different cuisines can make adjusted meal plans more enjoyable. Educational resources, cooking classes, and online tutorials can provide inspiration and build skills.

8. Flexibility:

No meal plan is set in stone. Life happens, and flexibility is key. If a meal doesn't work out, having a list of quick, safe backup options can help stay on track without stress.

9. Monitor and Adjust:

Keep a food diary to track how dietary changes affect well-being, energy levels, and health markers. Review and adjust meal plans as needed based on this feedback.

In Summary

Adjusting meal plans requires understanding individual needs, experimenting with substitutions, and being mindful of portion sizes and nutrient content. It's a process of learning and adaptation, aiming for a balance between meeting dietary requirements and enjoying meals. Always prioritize safety, especially when managing health conditions, and seek professional guidance to navigate dietary adjustments effectively.

6. Additional Resources

Managing Eating Out: Renal-Diet-Friendly Choices

Dining out or attending social gatherings while managing a renal diet can be challenging. However, with preparation and knowledge, you can make choices that align with your dietary needs. Here are some tips for navigating these situations:

1. Research and Plan Ahead:

- Check Menus Online: Many restaurants have their menus online. Look for dishes that are likely to fit within your dietary restrictions.
- Call Ahead: Don't hesitate to call the restaurant and ask about renal-friendly options or the possibility of customizing dishes to meet your needs.

2. Understand Menu Terms:

- Foods described as "grilled," "baked," or "steamed" are often better choices than those that are "fried," "breaded," or "creamy."
- Be cautious with terms like "au gratin," "parmigiana," "tempura," or "escalloped," as these often indicate high sodium or phosphorus content.

3. Make Special Requests:

- Don't be shy about asking for modifications. Requesting no added salt or sauce on the side can significantly impact the suitability of a dish.
- Ask for ingredients like cheese or nuts to be served on the side so you can control the amount.

4. Portion Control:

- Restaurant portions can be large. Consider sharing a dish with someone or asking for a half portion.
- You can also request a to-go box at the start of the meal and set aside part of your dish to help manage portion sizes.

5. Choose Beverages Wisely:

- Opt for water, unsweetened tea, or other low-potassium, low-phosphorus drinks. Avoid or limit alcoholic beverages and sodas, especially colas, which are high in phosphorus.

6. Managing Appetizers and Salads:

- Choose simple appetizers like a small salad with dressing on the side. Avoid salads with high-potassium ingredients or those loaded with cheese and nuts.
- Be mindful of soups, as they can be very high in sodium.

7. Navigating Main Courses:

- Look for lean protein options that are grilled or baked. Fish, chicken, and lean cuts of meat can be good choices if prepared simply.
- Be cautious with side dishes. Opt for steamed vegetables or a salad instead of fries or mashed potatoes, which may contain added dairy or salt.

8. Dessert Choices:

- If you choose to have dessert, look for simple options like fruit-based dishes. Be cautious of portion sizes and ingredients like chocolate or nuts, which may need to be limited on a renal diet.

9. Social Gatherings:

- Offer to bring a dish that you know fits within your dietary restrictions. This ensures there's something you can enjoy without worry.
- Focus on the social aspect rather than the food. Enjoy the company and conversation.

10. Stay Hydrated:

- Keep track of your fluid intake if you need to manage fluid restriction. Choosing water as your main drink can help avoid unintentional fluid overload.

Conclusion

Dining out and attending social events while following a renal diet requires a bit of foresight and assertiveness, but it can be a manageable and enjoyable part of your life. By making informed choices and requesting modifications when needed, you can maintain your dietary restrictions and enjoy a variety of culinary experiences.

Support and Motivation: Navigating the Journey with Others

Managing a health condition or adhering to a specific diet can feel isolating at times, but it's important to remember you're not alone. Finding support and motivation from the community, healthcare professionals, or support groups can significantly impact your journey. Here's how to connect with the support you need:

1. Leverage Healthcare Professionals:

- Dietitians and Nutritionists: These experts can provide personalized dietary advice, help you understand your nutritional needs, and offer practical tips for meal planning and preparation.
- Doctors and Nurses: Your healthcare team is there to support your overall health. They can answer medical questions and may be able to recommend support groups or other resources.
- Pharmacists: They can offer advice on medication management and how different prescriptions might affect your diet or health.

2. Connect with Support Groups:

- Local Support Groups: Many hospitals and community centers offer support groups for individuals with specific health conditions. These groups provide a space to share experiences, tips, and encouragement.
- Online Communities: Online forums and social media groups can be invaluable resources, offering support and advice from others who understand exactly what you're going through.
- National Organizations: Many national health organizations offer resources, including support groups, educational materials, and events.

3. Engage with Friends and Family:

- Share your journey with close friends and family members. They can offer emotional support, help with meal preparation, and accompany you to appointments or group meetings.
- Educate them about your dietary needs so they can be more accommodating during social gatherings or when dining out together.

4. Participate in Educational Workshops and Seminars:

- Many organizations and healthcare providers offer workshops on nutrition, lifestyle changes, and disease management. These can be great opportunities to learn and meet others with similar experiences.

5. Volunteer or Advocate:

- Getting involved in advocacy or volunteering for health-related causes can provide a sense of purpose and community. It's also a chance to educate others and make a difference in the broader conversation about health.

6. Set Realistic Goals:

- Work with your healthcare team to set achievable health and diet goals. Celebrate your milestones, no matter how small, to stay motivated.

7. Find a Motivation Buddy:

- Partner with someone who shares similar goals. Whether it's a friend, family member, or someone from a support group, checking in with each other can keep you both motivated.

8. Remember Self-Care:

- Managing a diet or health condition is just one part of your life. Make time for activities that you enjoy and that help you relax and de-stress.

9. Keep Learning:

- The more you know about your condition and how to manage it, the more empowered you'll feel. Stay curious and keep learning about new research, recipes, and strategies for living well.

Conclusion

Finding support is key to managing your health and dietary needs. Whether it's professional advice, the shared experiences of a support group, or the encouragement of friends and family, you don't have to navigate your journey alone. Surrounding yourself with a supportive network can provide the motivation and resilience needed to face challenges and celebrate successes on your path to wellness.

FAQs: Understanding the Renal Diet

What is a renal diet?

A renal diet is designed to support kidney function and slow the progression of kidney disease. It typically involves managing intake of sodium, potassium, phosphorus, proteins, and fluids to lessen the kidneys' workload and prevent waste buildup in the blood.

Why do I need to limit potassium on a renal diet?

Potassium is a mineral that, in high levels, can cause heart problems in people with kidney disease. Since damaged kidneys can't filter out excess potassium efficiently, it's important to manage its intake through diet.

How can I reduce sodium in my diet?

- Use herbs, spices, and lemon juice for flavor instead of salt.
- Choose fresh or frozen vegetables over canned ones, or rinse canned vegetables to remove some sodium.
- Avoid processed foods, fast foods, and cured meats, which are high in sodium.
- Read labels and choose products labeled "low-sodium" or "no salt added."

Why is phosphorus restricted in a renal diet?

Damaged kidneys can't remove excess phosphorus, leading to bone and cardiovascular problems. It's advised to limit foods high in phosphorus like dairy products, nuts, seeds, and processed foods, and to choose phosphorus binders if recommended by your healthcare provider.

How much protein should I eat?

Protein intake should be carefully managed on a renal diet. Too much can increase the kidneys' workload, but too little can lead to malnutrition. The right amount varies based on the stage of kidney disease, body size, and other health factors. It's best to consult with a dietitian.

Can I still eat out on a renal diet?

Yes, but it requires planning and modifications. Choose restaurants that offer fresh, made-to-order dishes. Request meals to be prepared without added salt and choose sides like steamed vegetables or salads (with dressing on the side) over higher sodium options.

How do I manage fluid intake?

Your healthcare provider may recommend a fluid restriction if your body is retaining fluid. Measure daily fluid intake, count fluids in foods like soups and ice cream, and use smaller cups to help control portions.

What about alcohol and caffeine?

Alcohol should be consumed in moderation, if at all, as it can affect blood pressure, alter kidney function, and add to fluid intake. Caffeine can also affect blood pressure and should be limited; opt for decaffeinated beverages.

How can I make sure I'm getting enough nutrients?

A balanced renal diet can meet most of your nutritional needs. However, due to restrictions, some people may need supplements for nutrients like vitamin D, calcium, or iron. It's essential to only take supplements recommended by your healthcare provider.

Is it necessary to see a dietitian?

Yes, a registered dietitian can create a personalized eating plan that meets your nutritional needs and food preferences while managing your kidney health. They can provide valuable guidance, support, and adjustments as your condition changes.

Conclusion

Adhering to a renal diet requires understanding your specific nutritional needs and how to manage them through diet and lifestyle changes. Consulting healthcare professionals and a registered dietitian is crucial in effectively managing kidney health and ensuring a balanced, nutritious diet that supports your overall well-being.

Embracing Your Journey on the Renal Diet

As we reach the conclusion of "Renal Diet for Beginners," it's important to reflect on the journey you've embarked upon. Navigating the complexities of a renal diet can seem daunting at first, but through understanding, patience, and commitment, it becomes a manageable and rewarding path toward preserving kidney health and enhancing overall well-being.

Embracing Adaptation

Adopting a renal diet necessitates changes in how you view food and nutrition. It's about making informed choices that support your kidneys while still enjoying delicious and nourishing meals. Remember, adaptation is key. As you become more familiar with your dietary needs, adjusting recipes and making smart food choices will become second nature.

Building Your Support System

You don't have to walk this path alone. Building a strong support system of healthcare professionals, dietitians, family, and friends can provide the encouragement and assistance you need. Support groups, whether in-person or online, can offer invaluable insights and camaraderie from those who truly understand your experiences.

Celebrating Small Victories

Every step you take towards managing your renal diet effectively is a victory worth celebrating. Whether it's successfully modifying a favorite recipe, learning to enjoy new foods, or noticing improvements in your health markers, acknowledge your progress. These accomplishments are milestones on your journey to better health.

Staying Informed and Flexible

The field of nutrition and kidney health is ever-evolving. Stay informed about the latest research and dietary recommendations by consulting with your healthcare team regularly. Being flexible and willing to adjust your diet as needed is crucial for managing kidney disease effectively.

Prioritizing Self-Care

Beyond diet, prioritizing overall self-care — including managing stress, staying active, and getting adequate rest — plays a crucial role in your health journey. Take time for activities that bring you joy and relaxation, as mental and emotional well-being is just as important as physical health.

Looking Forward

Looking forward, let this guide be a starting point for your continued exploration and mastery of the renal diet. The journey is not just about managing kidney disease; it's about living a full, healthy, and joyful life. Embrace the challenge, celebrate your resilience, and know that every choice you make in favor of your health is a step toward a brighter future.

Final Thoughts

As you close this chapter of your renal diet journey, remember that this is a journey of transformation and growth. With every meal, every choice, and every day, you are taking control of your health and steering it in a positive direction. The road may have its bumps and turns, but with knowledge, support, and determination, you can navigate it successfully.

May this book serve as a steadfast companion on your journey, providing you with the knowledge, recipes, and inspiration needed to thrive on your renal diet. Here's to your health, happiness, and a future filled with flavorful, kidney-friendly delights.

GET YOUR BONUS!

SCAN ME

OR COPY AND PAST

https://qrco.de/betsjB

Made in the USA
Columbia, SC
20 July 2024

39026379R10093